Tai Chi Therapy

THE SCIENCE OF METAROBICS®

For Cancer, Heart & Lung Disease, Asthma, Diabetes, Immunity, Pain & Healthy Living

Pete Gryffin, PhD, MS

NOTE TO READERS
This publication is based on research, but in a new and emerging area. The ideas and thoughts presented in this publication are the opinions and views of the author. It is meant to provide helpful information to bring greater awareness to potential exercises for health. This publication is provided and sold solely for educational purposes, and is not meant to be used as a substitute for medical advice or professional health services. It is recommended that the reader should consult with his or her medical provider, or other professional service, before using or trying any of the practices discussed in this publication, or changing current health practices. The author and publisher specifically disclaim all responsibility for any liability, loss of risk, personal or otherwise, which is incurred as a consequence, directly or indirectly, of the use and application of any of the contents of this book.

Copyright © 2014 by Peter A. Gryffin

Photo Credits:
Page 31 Photo courtesy of Keith Van Sickle, used with permission. All other photos by Lee Gryffin.

All rights reserved. No part of this publication may be reproduced, stored in a retrieval system, or transmitted in any form or by any means, electronic, photocopying, recording, or otherwise without the prior written permission of the author. For information and permissions, e-mail: drgryffin@metarobics.com

For more information or to book an event or speaking engagement, contact Dr. Gryffin at *Metarobics.com* or e-mail: drgryffin@metarobics.com

TAI CHI THERAPY

THE SCIENCE OF METAROBICS®

Contents

Preface   i

Chapter 1: Metarobics and Tai Chi Therapy
A New Paradigm of Fitness
*How a Student with Cancer Changed
my Understanding of Health*   1

Chapter 2: Qi - Science or Magic?
*Experiences with Language
and the Mysteries of Qi*   23

Chapter 3: Metarobics and Cancer
*The Battle against Hypoxia (Oxygen Deficiency)
and the Experiences of Three Students
with Cancer*   36

Chapter 4: Metarobics - Heart Disease,
Stroke and Kidney Disease
Dealing with the Pressures of Life   50

Chapter 5: Metarobics and Lung Disease
(COPD and Asthma)
Better Breathing through Tai Chi and Qi Gong   72

Chapter 6: Metarobics for Immunity,
Diabetes, and Pain
Enhancing Qualify of Life   81

Chapter 7: Essential Elements of
Metarobics and Tai Chi for Therapy
Teaching, Learning, and Researching
Tai Chi and Qi Gong for Health   101

Conclusion and Future Directions
Metarobics and Tai Chi Therapy
The Beginning of a New Field of Exercise   127

References   143

Preface

Over the past 15 years of teaching Tai Chi, I have heard remarkable stories from students regarding benefits for health. Health concerns can be a driving force for starting Tai Chi. Indeed many of those teaching Tai Chi today began practice as the result of a diagnosis with a life threatening condition, in a desperate last ditch effort to avoid death. And it worked, with sometimes miraculous and dramatic effects. Several of the case stories in this book are from those teachers, and their stories are powerful and moving.

Tai Chi has been studied by researchers for almost every health condition out there – from heart, lung and kidney disease, to cancer, stroke, diabetes, asthma, Alzheimer's, multiple sclerosis, chronic pain, immunity and more. Much of that research is presented in this book, along with over 50 case stories from those who have directly experienced the benefits of Tai Chi. But what was missing in the research was *why* these exercises were having such benefits. *Chapter Two – Qi: Science or Magic?* details views from a Traditional Chinese Medicine and cultural perspective. However little has been done to understand how and why exercises such as Tai Chi were having benefits from a physiological perspective.

Following the change in condition of three of my students with cancer (one quite dramatic), I realized that there must be a physiological and measureable response which would explain these results. My research revealed a link between hypoxia (reduction of oxygen reaching various tissues or areas of the body) and enhanced blood oxygen saturation, diffusion and metabolic function. A mechanism of health distinctly different from that of aerobic and anaerobic exercise.

I then realized this meant that a third and new school of fitness needed to be developed. One which could explain why and how exercises which are neither aerobic nor strength based were having such dramatic benefits for health. Indeed, it has been noted that Tai Chi has no aerobic specific effects, in an extensive review of Tai Chi studies.[1] Yet Tai Chi has been found to have benefits for a wide range of chronic conditions. So if Tai Chi and related exercises are not aerobic exercises, then what are they? Since measurements suggest a positive effect on oxygen based metabolism, I coined the word *Metarobics*.

Metarobic exercise is a good fit with Aerobic and Anaerobic categories of exercise. As detailed in the first chapter of this book, aerobic exercise results in either no change to a drop in blood oxygen saturation and diffusion, depending on intensity. Exercises such as Tai Chi enhance blood oxygen saturation and diffusion. As a new theory, Metarobics explains how and why exercises such as Tai Chi can benefit such a wide range of chronic conditions. It turns out that relaxing the body in conjunction with slow abdominal breathing is not just good for your health, but fantastic!

Tai Chi Therapy: The New Science of Metarobics, is a unique book from many perspectives. Aside from documenting and presenting theories and research for a new category of exercise, I have included life changing testimonials and stories. These stories are many and dramatic, so much so that I have created a section on

Metarobics.com to post the growing number of accounts. Some are accounts which were personally related to me, others are from various books and websites (listed in the references).

Chapters one and two present research supporting that exercises such as Tai Chi enhance blood oxygen saturation, diffusion and oxygen based metabolism, as an effect unique from other forms of exercise. Chapter three continues with research specific to cancer, which is what prompted many of my original observations. Chapters four, five and six document research and theoretical effects for a wide range of other conditions, including heart and lung disease, stroke, kidney disease, asthma, diabetes, immunity and chronic pain.

Although the stories and research presented in this book affirms the live giving benefits people have derived from forms of Tai Chi and related exercises, it should be noted that there are many styles and methods of teaching. Before choosing a school or teacher, you are encouraged to read *Chapter Seven: Essential Elements of Metarobics and Tai Chi for Therapy*. It is also important to discuss any changes in health routines with your doctor.

The conclusion summarizes the current state of Metarobics as a new field of exercise, as well as psychological benefits of Tai Chi as a form of moving meditation and mindfulness based practice (including uses for smoking cessation and other addictive behaviors). Research related to Alzheimer's and Parkinson's is also presented, as well as implications related to exercises which do not necessarily fit the typical category of aerobic or anaerobic forms of exercise, such as walking and yoga. Over time Metarobics may come to include a wide variety of exercises.

Many people already practice some form of these exercises in various parts of the world, including the

United States. It is my hope that this book will help an even greater number of people understand and benefit from these exercises. People ran, swam and bicycled before Dr. Ken Cooper came out with his book Aerobics[2] in 1968, but it took his work to document the unique physiological effects of these exercises, leading to the diversity and growth of aerobic exercises that we have today. Metarobics does the same thing for Tai Chi and forms of Qi Gong, and may come to embrace a wide variety of exercises which do not quite fit conventional categories. Enjoy the book, and with a greater understanding of Metarobics, I encourage you to research your local opportunities, and check out the resources available on Metarobics.com.

Dr. Pete Gryffin

Chapter One

METAROBICS® and Tai Chi Therapy

The Evolution of a New Paradigm of Health and Fitness

How a Student with Cancer Changed my Understanding of Exercise

My awareness of how the body responds to certain kinds of movement occurred over a period of several years, and quite by accident. It was a gradual process (detailed in the following chapters), beginning with the first student who came to me convinced that Tai Chi had cured her cancer. Over time, I came to realize that a large variety of chronic diseases shared a common element. An element directly affected by Tai Chi and similar exercises, which have unique and measurable effects on blood oxygen saturation and

At Death's Door

"The doctors had tried everything – chemotherapy, radiation, nothing seemed to work. All that happened was that my hair fell out, and I was in constant pain. I was taking five of the maximum doses of pain pills daily, but with little effect. Then a friend told me they read about a guy with brain cancer being cured by an exercise called Tai Chi. By the time I learned about Tai Chi, my doctor told me I had about three weeks left to live. Not ready to give up, I looked for a class and found one at the community college. The teacher made me a video that night, which would talk me through the form. A little over a week later, I was completely off of pain pills. If nothing else, that was worth it. And although I am still battling cancer, three weeks has come and gone, and two years later I am still alive."

– Karen (*Personal Account*).

(Throughout this book I present case stories highlighting the healing benefits of Tai Chi. Some stories may be paraphrased for length, focusing on highlighted benefits. As inspirational as many of these stories can be, always consult with your doctor regarding any changes to your health care).

---

diffusion. It is worth noting that hypoxia (reduction of oxygen reaching various tissues or areas of the body) underlies the majority of chronic diseases plaguing society, including cancer, heart, lung and kidney disease, stroke and diabetes. Hypoxia is also implicated in asthma, chronic pain and immunity.

My research and experiences consistently supported that many of the health benefits of Tai Chi and forms of Qi Gong (breathing exercises) had to be the result of a physiological response related to enhanced blood oxygen saturation and diffusion, a mechanism which was distinctly different from aerobic and anaerobic forms exercise. A mechanism with direct and beneficial effects on hypoxia. By default, this meant that a third and "new" category of exercise must exist. My research and observations pointed to a dynamic state of relaxation and enhanced respiration as underlying the primary mechanism of action. This "Third School of Fitness," which I call Metarobics for reasons described below, will be developed out of the slow movements of Tai Chi, as well as forms of Yoga and Qi Gong when focused on relaxation and the breath.

Everyone knows that exercise is good for your health. It can enhance strength, cardiovascular health and even mental health. Yet even highly fit people still get sick, experience degenerative diseases of the bones, joints and organs, and are subject to cancer and many other ills (albeit less than their sedentary counterparts). Based on a growing body of research and testimonies from those who have benefited from Tai Chi, Metarobic exercises may add another component. Metarobic exercises enhance fitness at the cellular level, which in conjunction with a healthy diet and other forms of exercise, could supply the missing element in total health and immunity, to make a person as free from illness, degenerative disease and cancer as it is possible to get.

These exercises have profound health effects for many conditions (documented throughout this book), yet as an exercise they are not fast paced enough to be considered truly aerobic (some Qi Gong movements and standing Yoga poses are stationary, with a focus on slow relaxed breathing). Neither do they work the large muscle groups the way strength training does. Tai Chi is sometimes categorized as a "low to moderate" aerobic exercise, particularly if you "up" the intensity. However, focusing on speeding up the movements of Tai Chi in an attempt to make it a form of aerobic exercise may negate some of the benefits unique to totally relaxing the body through slow movement.

A Miracle, or Tai Chi?

"After I retired, I ended up getting rheumatoid arthritis which developed rapidly. The doctor said before long I would be unable to walk, and would need a wheelchair. By the time I heard about Tai Chi, I could barely stand on my own. I began practicing every day, doing Tai Chi in my wheel chair, and soon I could do it standing. The doctor was surprised at how much progress I made in less than six months after starting Tai Chi. He was dubious about Tai Chi, but said to keep with it. I am glad I did, because before two years had passed, I was pain free and able to walk on my own. I completely recovered my former health and mobility, maybe even more so. Seeing the changes in my body, the rheumatologist was calling it a miracle. Maybe it was – the miracle of Tai Chi."

– Elisa Morella (From *Tai Chi for Health Institute Newsletter*)

From an intuitive perspective, that such a wide range of health benefits are being attributed to these forms of exercise, it seems likely that something unique is going on in the body. My research supports this, and sheds light on what will become a whole new field of exercise. Fifty or so years ago running was almost the sole domain of track and field, and the concept of running for your health was considered unusual. I can recall stories of people running along city streets who would be asked jokingly "what are you running from?" The rapid gyrations of modern aerobic programs could have gotten one committed to an asylum. It wasn't until 1968, with the release of the ground breaking book *Aerobics*[1] by Dr. Kenneth Cooper, that the concept of aerobic health was popularized, along with a new word for a new form of exercise.

Dr. Cooper noted that those with large developed muscles from body building exhibited poor performance in running, swimming and cycling. From these observations of differences between runners and weightlifters, he coined the term aerobics, and founded a new field of health. Now there are few who are not aware of how important it is to perform some form of aerobic exercise, at least a few days every week. It would be easy to assume that our current understanding of aerobics is fairly well established – it is now a multi-billion dollar industry, and is a well-established field of study within the health and kinesiology departments of many universities. It is easy to assume that we now know everything there is to know about the body and how it works, so much so that it is equally easy to make assumptions that movement is movement is movement.

But as far as alternative forms of exercise go, there are still new frontiers and ways of moving for health and fitness. Current research on alternative forms of health and fitness such as Tai Chi and forms of Qi Gong are primarily oriented around the benefits of these exercises, with little in the way of how or why these exercises provide benefits. In research on the benefits of Tai Chi and Qi Gong, often no reason is given for the benefits for various conditions. Alternatively, benefits may be attributed to a vague concept of "Qi" as "Vital Energy," or as a mystical force (which is further discussed in Chapter Two: Qi – Science or Magic?). As long as these exercises result in measurable benefits, it may seem of little matter as to why or how the benefits of these exercises are derived. But a greater understanding of the physiological mechanisms involved will help to better research, promote and understand a growing field of health and fitness.

In a collaborative overview of the unique differences between Tai Chi and similar exercises, Doctors Linda Larkey, Roger Jahnke, Jennifer Etnier and Julie Gonzalez,[2] noted that what differentiates Tai Chi and related exercises from conventional forms of exercise is a focus of the mind on the body, while using breathing as a vehicle for deep relaxation. The authors note that based on differences from aerobic exercises, a new category of exercise needs to be defined, one involving meditative movement.

From Immobility to Freedom

"I was diagnosed with peripheral neuropathy and told that there was nothing to be done ... just inevitable immobility. I was barely able to walk, and had difficulty getting in and out of a chair, was chronically fatigued, depressed, and despite pain meds, continued to have intense cramping in my arms and legs at night. I found it impossible to do much of anything. Then I was introduced to Tai Chi, and began practicing regularly. 1 year later I was able to walk completely unaided, except for a walking stick. My blood pressure and cholesterol/triglyceride levels were within normal limits. My blood pressure medicine was cut in half by my physician four months after starting Tai Chi. I have no more chronic fatigue, and sleep well at night with little or no cramping. My balance has improved; I walk faster and more evenly ... I no longer use a cane. I can get up from most chairs easily. A year into practicing Tai Chi and I am a much healthier and yes, a much happier person."

– Saundra (Posted in *Tai Chi for Everyone*).

It is for this reason that I coined the term Metarobics (*alt. Metaerobics*), as forms of movement distinct from aerobic and anaerobic modes of exercise. The theory of Metarobics is centered on the unique way the body responds in relationship to oxygen use in the body during slow relaxed movements. I use the word Metarobics for two primary reasons. The first is due to measurements which show that slow relaxed movements, coupled with deep abdominal breathing, maximizes blood oxygen saturation and diffusion to every cell of the body. With the root of "Meta" as "Above." Metarobics thus becomes "Above Aerobics," as an enhanced way of using oxygen in the body.

Neither strength training nor cardiovascular in the traditional sense, Metarobics is a very different way of moving distinct from traditional exercise, affecting the body in ways as novel as aerobics differs from strength training. This does not discount the benefits of aerobic exercise and strength training, which are still necessary for a healthy life. But it may point to an additional medium of exercise which can enhance current activities and total health, or provide a form of exercise for those unable to participate in more vigorous activities.

The second reason Metarobics is a good term for these exercises relates to preliminary research (documented throughout this book) which indicates that enhanced blood oxygen saturation and diffusion enhances metabolic function, to optimize cellular functioning and health. In this case, the word Metarobics relates to enhanced oxygen based metabolism. When you engage in aerobic or anaerobic exercise, the large muscle groups command the supply of oxygen in the body. This is considered the primary reason why you get stomach cramps if you eat before intense exercise (as the blood is drawn from the organs and is redirected to the muscles). It is worth noting that cancer is almost unknown in the oxygen rich environment of the large muscle groups[3] (see Chapter Three: Tai Chi and Cancer).

My research indicates that the following two factors lie behind many if not most of the remarkable benefits of Tai Chi and similar exercises. Research supports that the following two factors may affect a wide variety of physiological responses in the body (including production of proteins and amino acids involved in metabolic function):[4]

1) **Reduced muscle tension, combined with slow full breaths, results in greater blood flow and oxygen distribution throughout the entire body (including the organs), as opposed to more vigorous forms of exercise which result in blood flow being redirected to the large muscle groups.**

2) **Increased blood oxygen saturation and diffusion results in, or is an indication of, enhanced metabolic function, with a resultant increase in the disease fighting and healing abilities of the body.**

Measurable increases in blood oxygen saturation and diffusion during Metarobic exercise indicates that if enhanced blood oxygen saturation is not directly the cause of the many benefits attributed to these exercises, it is at least an indication that something unique is going on in the body. Something different from conventional exercise, which results in no change or even a drop in blood oxygen saturation (depending on intensity – see the tables on pages 17-18). If not a direct cause of benefits, the increase may be linked to a "surplus" resulting from more efficient oxygen use and diffusion in the body. Or it may be a combination of increased blood oxygen saturation and diffusion, enhanced oxygen based metabolism, and other factors yet to be determined.

The research presented in this book supports the observation that exercises such a Tai Chi, and forms of Yoga and Qi Gong which focus on relaxation and the breath, have distinct mechanisms of benefit unique from conventional exercise. Time and further research will help establish a greater understanding of the mechanisms involved with Metarobic exercises, beginning with the foundation presented in this book. The many studies presented, which implicate hypoxia (the reduction of oxygen reaching various tissues or areas of the body) in a wide range of chronic conditions, indicates that the theory of Metarobics is on the right track.

RESULTS OF MEASUREMENTS DURING TAI CHI AND OTHER EXERCISES

In a series of studies documenting the effects of Tai Chi on blood oxygen saturation, compared to conventional exercise, Tai Chi practice resulted in a significant increase of one to three percentage points. Walking resulted in no significant change, while vigorous forms of exercise resulted in a drop in blood oxygen saturation of up to six percentage points or more.[5] The more vigorous the exercise, the greater the drop. A one to three percentage point increase may not sound like much, but considering that a typical range for blood oxygen saturation is 95 to 99 percent, even one percentage point is a 25 percent increase in this range.

Blood oxygen saturation refers to the amount of oxygen carried by arterial blood, and can be measured using a pulse oximeter. Blood is oxygenated in the lungs, as oxygen molecules are transferred into the blood stream. According to the Mayo Clinic,[6] if blood oxygen levels are low (below 90 to 95 percent), the body cannot function properly, resulting in hypoxemia, shortness of breath and high blood pressure. Chronically low levels of blood oxygen saturation below 90% can result in death. Blood oxygen saturation level is one of the standard measures taken in emergency rooms, along with pulse and blood pressure.

Ongoing hypoxemia can result in shortness of breath and high blood pressure. It also has a higher association with the development of cancer, according to a growing body of research which is presented in Chapter Three: *Metarobics and Cancer*. Hypoxemia, or low blood oxygen saturation, can affect a number of conditions. Dr. Chenchen Wang, a researcher at Tufts Medical Center, conducted a review of 57 studies and 34 case series on the use of hyperbaric oxygen for wound treatment.[7]

Hyperbaric oxygen therapy is based on the premise that raising tissue oxygen levels will enhance the natural wound healing ability of the body. Dr. Wang and colleagues noted that wounds tend to have a reduced oxygen supply (hypoxia), which makes it difficult for the body to heal wounds. Aside from wound treatment, hyperbaric oxygen therapy has also been used to treat gangrene, infections and radiation injuries (which may account for why Tai Chi may have helped Karen with her radiation therapy).

Studies on the effects of hypoxia and hypoxemia support that slow moving exercises such as Tai Chi (and forms of Qi Gong and Yoga which focus on relaxation and the breath) may be a vital element in health, as well as in the prevention of disease. Relaxation and a focus on the breath may be a key component, as indicated by the case story below. Forms of Tai Chi, Yoga and Qi Gong which involve faster paces, or a focus on strength, may not yield the same benefits.

Breath Focused Yoga for a Drug Free Life

I was active (running, weight lifting and another yoga practice) but still had chronic issues with asthma and high blood pressure. I thought I'd gotten all the benefits I could from exercise. Then I began a form of Yoga with a focus on breathing exercises. At that time I was using 2 medications for my blood pressure and 4 daily medications just to control my asthma (6 during bad periods). As I've very slowly progressed in my practice, I've been able to drop medications gradually, with the supervision of my physician of course. First one blood pressure medication, then the second. Now I'm off all my asthma drugs, including the rescue inhaler. This morning I ran with no asthma medication for the first time ever. I can't tell you how good that felt. I'm feeling great, minus the thousands of dollars of drugs I needed just six months ago.

– Margaret (From *Bikram Yoga St. Louis*)

Research related to an increase in blood oxygen saturation is but the first step. Possibly an important one, based on the implications of hypoxia in many chronic conditions, presented in the following chapters, and the central role of Qi (or "Air" as literally translated)[8] in the attributions of health benefits from a traditional Chinese perspective (the importance of which is discussed in the next chapter).

STUDIES ON THE EFFECTS OF TAI CHI ON BLOOD OXGYEN SATURATION

As mentioned above, aerobic forms of exercise consistently result in a drop of blood oxygen saturation ranging from one to six points, depending on intensity. In a study on the effects of walking on blood oxygen saturation, over 200 individuals were tested during a six minute walk test. No significant changes were found in either direction.[9] Another study on the effects of high intensity exercise found an average drop of 2.9 percentage points during cycling, and a 4.9 percentage point drop during running in endurance athletes.[10]

But what of the effects of exercises such as Tai Chi on blood oxygen saturation, which focus specifically on relaxation, the breath, and enhancing oxygen use in the body? The next step was to measure those who practiced Tai Chi. The blood oxygen saturation of 31 Tai Chi practitioners was measured during the practice of Tai Chi, using a fingertip pulse oximeter (a small electronic device which measures blood oxygen saturation).[5] Measurements were taken during the "grasp the bird's tail," "brush knee, twist step," and the "part the horse's mane" sections of the Yang style Tai Chi form (considered one of the most representative as a slow paced style of Tai Chi).

The three sections above where chosen due to the focus on relaxation. Later measurements confirmed that the kicking section, repulse the monkey (involving lifting one leg into the air) and movements which include sinking down to the ground (such as "snake creeps down") do not result in the same degree of increase in blood oxygen saturation. The differences and implications related to variance of movements is discussed later in this book.

No Bones About It, Tai Chi Restored My Health

"I began Tai Chi six years ago due to osteoporosis. I swam regularly, but using weights was out of the question, and my walking was limited. Then I started Tai Chi. My bone density is back to normal, and I can now do so much more, thanks to Tai Chi."

– Carol (*Tai Chi for Health Institute Newsletters*).

The study included students with a mix of experience, ranging from less than two months to a period of several years, with the exception of three participants, who had been practicing Tai Chi for five to 15 years. The average increase in blood oxygen saturation in the 31 participants was 1.29 points, with a zero to three point range (three of the students who had been practicing for less than two months had no significant change in blood oxygen saturation).[5] I later had the opportunity to measure eight practitioners in an ongoing senior Tai Chi class. All participants in this class had been practicing Tai Chi between 10 to 40 years. This group exhibited a 1.92 average increase during Tai Chi, with scores again ranging from a one to three point increase from resting levels before Tai Chi.

Following these measurements, I began to wonder if the three students in the first study, who had no change in oxygen saturation levels, might be due to not knowing the form, since they had just started the class. During the initial learning phase trying to memorize and figure out movements might not permit levels of relaxation or breath-work necessary to reduce muscle tension and enhance oxygen saturation and diffusion.

Would a person who had never practiced Tai Chi get similar benefits from following a simplified section of the Tai Chi form with no learning curve, with a focus on relaxation and the breath? Recruiting a participant who was a regular runner (to compare oxygen saturation during running as well as Tai Chi), I conducted a repeated measures study. This form of study can use a single individual by taking repeated measures, to evaluate an intervention for significant effects. It would be the equivalent of measuring one person 30 times, or 30 people once. This format also has the benefit of controlling for differences between individuals.

His average resting blood oxygen saturation level was 96.25, with a resting heart rate of 68 beats per minute. Running on a treadmill at a moderate aerobic intensity increased his heart rate to an average of 133 beats per minute, and resulted in a drop in blood oxygen saturation to an average of 95.83 percent. However, when following the "grasp the bird's tail" section of the Tai Chi form, with verbal cues and a focus on relaxation and the breath, his blood oxygen saturation level increased to an average of 97.22 percent. His average heart rate during the "grasp the bird's tail" section was 96.2 beats per minute.

I then conducted a series of measurements using a variety of exercises, including "Qi Walking" (using Tai Chi principles during walking), in a 50 year old healthy male. This individual had practiced Tai Chi and Qi Gong for approximately 45 minutes almost daily for over 20 years, and had been running one to two miles, three to four times a week, for about three years. During these measurements, I was able to continuously monitor blood oxygen saturation throughout the entire 108 Yang form, to get an overall average for heart rate and blood oxygen saturation.

Measurements showed the highest increase occurred during the "grasp the bird's tail" section. In over a hundred measurements during Tai Chi practice, results were the same. Average blood oxygen saturation increased by one to three points, depending on the movement. During more strenuous movements, such as the kicking section and "snake creeps down" there is either no increase in blood oxygen saturation, or only a mild increase.

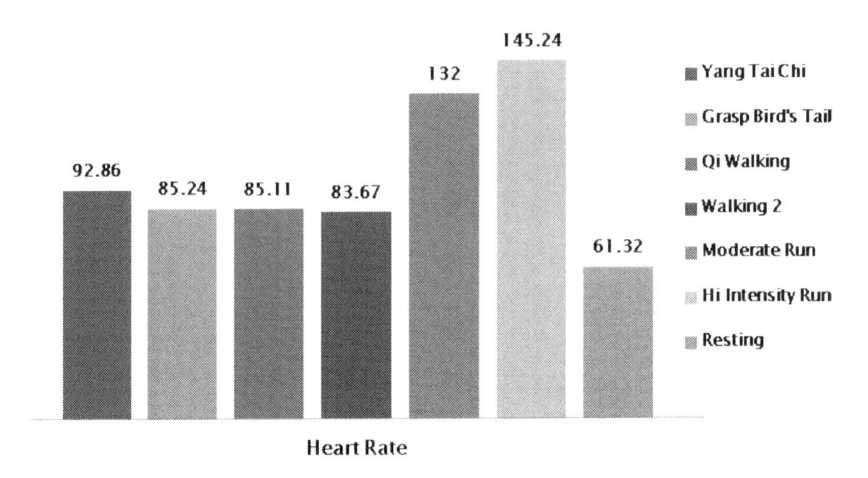

Heart Rate

- Yang Tai Chi: 92.86
- Grasp Bird's Tail: 85.24
- Qi Walking: 85.11
- Walking 2: 83.67
- Moderate Run: 132
- Hi Intensity Run: 145.24
- Resting: 61.32

Heart Rate for 50 year old subject. Heart rate for Yang Tai Chi is the average heart rate across all movements, including kicking and sinking down on one leg (such as "snake creeps down"). Grasp the Bird's Tail is a stationary series of movements in Tai Chi, involving shifting of weight, but no stepping. Walking2 is regular walking, as opposed to Qi Walking, which involves focus on relaxation, deeper coordinated breathing, and maximizing body dynamics during walking.

Normal walking resulted in a mild but statistically non-significant increase (with a range of readings both below and above his resting blood oxygen saturation levels). But when the principles of relaxation, efficiency of movement and deep breathing where applied while walking, effects where experienced similar to Tai Chi and Qi Gong exercises, with an increase during all measurements. The following tables present heart rate and blood oxygen saturation during various exercises, including Tai

Chi movements, Qi Walking, regular walking, moderate and high intensity running, and compareison to resting levels.

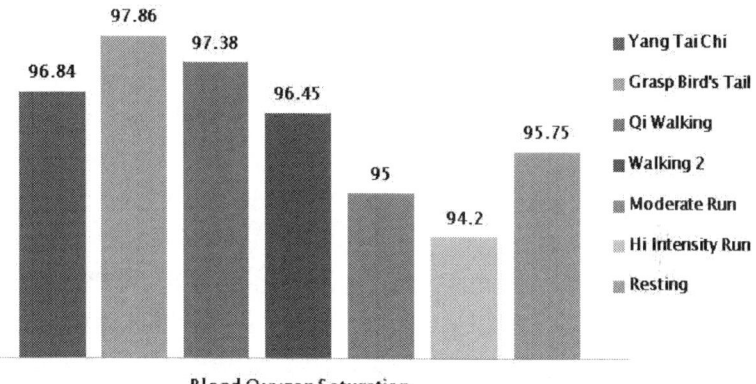

Blood Oxygen Saturation

- Yang Tai Chi: 96.84
- Grasp Bird's Tail: 97.86
- Qi Walking: 97.38
- Walking 2: 96.45
- Moderate Run: 95
- Hi Intensity Run: 94.2
- Resting: 95.75

Blood Oxygen Saturation (SpO2) for 50 year old subject. Yang Tai Chi is the average across all movements, including kicking and sinking down on one leg (such as "snake creeps down"). Grasp the Bird's Tail is a stationary series of movements in Tai Chi, involving shifting of weight, but no stepping. Walking2 is regular walking, as opposed to Qi Walking, which involves focus on relaxation, deeper coordinated breathing, and maximizing body dynamics during walking.

Those forms of exercise focusing on relaxation, efficient movement and slow deep breathing yielded consistently higher blood oxygen saturation. It is also important to note that heart rate during Tai Chi and related exercises did not approach levels considered necessary for aerobic benefits, being in the "warm up/cool down" phase. Yet many and often dramatic benefits for health have been reported for these exercises, documented in the following chapters.

Based on these measurements and Metarobic theory, I then developed an even easier to follow format of Tai Chi which consisted of shifting the feet back and forth in place, through the range of movements in Tai Chi (not including the kicking section, or the movement "snake creeps down"). My teacher mentioned that a similar format was used by political prisoners who knew Tai Chi, when space was limited, by switching steps in place. He jokingly called this "Jail Cell" style Tai Chi. This format maximized relaxation and movement to the point that blood oxygen saturation remained elevated throughout the form. Further study would be needed, to determine if more strenuous movements during the traditional form help with blood diffusion through increased internal pressure, or have other desirable benefits.

Pa Duan Jin (literally the "eight pieces of silk brocade," and also called the "eight treasures," due to its many health benefits) is a Qi Gong exercise which alternates standing and bent kneed poses while moving the upper body through a gentle range of stationary motions. During the standing poses, blood oxygen saturation typically rises two points or so. But during the bent kneed poses, blood oxygen saturation typically increases only one point from resting. Again, the question needs to be asked, are there unique benefits which might be derived from the bent kneed poses, beyond stronger knees and legs?

Benefits during the kicking section and other parts of the Tai Chi form, which may not be oxygen specific, include the development of enhanced balance. Tai Chi has proven effective for developing balance, which is a valuable benefit, particularly as one grows older. Death from falls is the leading cause of accidental death in older adults.[12] So aside from Metarobic benefits resulting from slow relaxed movements with a focus on the breath, it should also be kept in mind that there are many auxiliary benefits, including psychological benefits related to mindfulness, addiction and stress reduction (discussed in the conclusion).

Drugs for Life, or Tai Chi?

"I suffered from a lot of pain as a result of various sports injuries over the years. I was suffering from shoulder and neck pain, as well as pain in my right hip. I was also suffering from bone problems and inflammation. My doctor had told me that I had osteoarthritis in my neck, and that I would have to take anti-inflammatory drugs for the rest of my life. Since doing Tai Chi, I do not have pain anymore, and do not need to take those drugs. After practicing Tai Chi for six years everything has gotten better."

– Solange, (From *Sing Ong Tai Chi*)

The observations and research I have made over the past 10 years provides a much needed physiological theory behind the benefits of exercises such as Tai Chi and forms of Qi Gong. Physiological mechanisms which can be measured, tested and validated. Although enhanced blood oxygen saturation and diffusion may not explain all of the beneficial effects of Metarobic exercises, if nothing else, it is a valuable starting point. One which provides a better understanding for more effective practice, research and promotion of Metarobic based exercises.

Understanding of physiological mechanisms behind the benefits of Tai Chi, Qi Gong, forms of Yoga and other Metarobic exercises, does not invalidate anyone looking for the mysterious, but it does offer a scientific explanation for why many of the benefits result, and can help to maximize practice for optimal effect. Practitioners of forms of Tai Chi, Yoga and Qi Gong have reported benefits similar to many medications taken to relieve chronic pain and inflammation,[13-16] but without the severe side effects (side effects with can include heart attack, stroke, skin and allergic reactions, ulcers and death). One should never stop taking or alter medications prescribed by your doctor, but if these exercises can have effects similar to drugs, but without the adverse side effects, it is worth discussing with your doctor how to best integrate Tai Chi or other Metarobic exercises as a complementary exercise.

Behavioral aspects of health is becoming a growing field, as people realize more and more how much our negative behaviors impact health and quality of life. Indeed, according the Center for Disease Control (CDC), seven out of ten causes of early deaths are preventable through lifestyle changes.[12] Metarobics offers a simple avenue to add a new dimension to life which can reduce stress, enhance sleep, and help your body to function more efficiently to combat a wide variety of ills. Although not a complete fix for the need of a balanced diet and a complete exercise regimen (which also benefits from cardiovascular, strength, and stretching exercises), Metarobics adds a new dimension and way to enhance health, particularly for those who are limited in their ability to exercise.

Chapter Two

Qi – Science or Magic?

*Experiences with Language
and the Mysteries of Qi*

Tai Chi and similar exercises are yielding phenomenal results for a large variety of health concerns. When I began collecting case stories for this book, I was amazed at the number of people who have benefited from these exercises in often dramatic ways. That Tai Chi and various Qi Gong exercises increase blood oxygen saturation indicates that it is no coincidence that the Chinese word "Qi" (pronounced "Chi") is so strongly associated with these exercises. Despite Qi's common association with the metaphysical and energy work, at its most basic level Qi is best understood from its literal translation as "Air."

Pacemaker Free Through Tai Chi

I had to have a pacemaker due to Bradycardia. I was told that I would need a pacemaker the rest of my life. I became depressed, gave up running, and began using anti-depressants. I year later I decided to try Tai Chi. Initially I could barely finish a class, but within two months I noticed improvements. I returned to my cardiologist, and was told that my heart was now regulating normally, and that I no longer needed the pacemaker. I am now off of all medications for depression and hyper-tension as well. I am also now running again.

– Ted. (*Personal Account*).

The Chinese word Qi, as listed in most Chinese-English dictionaries (such as the Oxford Chinese Dictionary[1]) is directly translated as "Air." Some Chinese-English dictionaries take into account cultural aspects of the language (one dictionary even stated that the concept of Qi is so unique to Chinese culture that it cannot be translated).[2] This brings us back to the question of Qi, which is the basic attribution behind the benefits of exercises such as Tai Chi and Qi Gong. In Traditional Chinese Medicine, and much of the Tai Chi community, the word Qi is typically translated as "Vital Energy."[3] Vital Energy is a rather vague term, but does however reflect the role of oxygen based metabolism in all of the functions of the body, from thinking, digesting, movement, and even in healing and physical repair of the body. Tai Chi is considered a form of "Qi Gong," due to its slow movements and the deep breathing component. Qi Gong, with "air" as the root of Qi, and Gong as "cultivation" or "work," can be translated as "Breath Cultivation," "Breath Work," or even "Breathing Exercise." As such, Qi Gong can include a wide variety of exercises.

Tai Chi – A "Mind-Body Prescription for Cancer."

"I had been diagnosed with a very aggressive form of Thyroid Cancer two years earlier, and had just received very bad news. The cancer had come back and my prognosis was not a good one. Thyroid cancer has the reputation of being the "good cancer" because it is often curable. Something like 93% of all thyroid cancers are cured with surgery and a radioactive iodine pill. Unfortunately, this leaves 7% of us without a cure and with a lot of anxiety. After my 4th surgery I was told that I would need aggressive beam radiation to my neck, and would need chemotherapy to make the radiation more effective. I don't think I was ever as nervous or scared in my life. Wandering the halls of the Dana-Farber Cancer Institute, I saw a flyer that mentioned a Tai Chi/Qi Gong class. I knew that most things related to the cancer were out of my control, but I had the feeling that doing something that I did have control over might be helpful. All through my difficult treatments I looked forward to doing the "Mind-Body Prescription" daily. I know that it helped me deal with fatigue, pain, muscle atrophy, and much, much more."

– Rick (From *Tai Chi and Qi Gong for Health and Wellness*).

The realization of the literal translation of Qi was one of the occurrences which prompted my understanding that efficient oxygen use was important for the health of the body. Despite its literal translation, over the years, the word Qi has come to be used for everything from "vital energy," as mentioned above, to being described as a "mystical force which permeates the universe."[4] Qi is frequently relegated to the same mystical realm as the "force" of Star Wars fame. It wasn't until my experience teaching English at a Chinese school, that I realized that the basic Chinese view of Qi is entirely different from common perceptions based on movies and myth. One that has severe implications for a new field of health and fitness.

While teaching English at the Chinese school, I used the word Qi as an example for something relating to the spirit. The class met my comments with confused looks, so I asked what it was that confused them. It turned out to be the word Qi, which to the class simply meant "Air" or "Oxygen." It would be like mistaking oxygen for the word spirit, and saying to a group of young Catholics; "In the name of the Father, the Son, and the Holy Oxygen."

The students in the class elaborated on the word Qi, including a point that I had been dimly aware of, but only now realized was particularly significant. The Chinese character for Qi represents steam, or air, rising from cooked rice. I looked in a Chinese-English dictionary, and sure enough, the first definition of the word Qi was air.

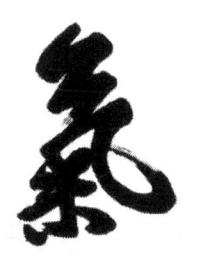

The symbol for Qi (Chi), represented by steam rising from cooked rice.[5]

    The next time I met with my Chinese Tai Chi teacher, I asked about this concept of Qi as simply "air" or "oxygen." He explained that in most cases, Qi does simply mean the air we breathe, but occasionally it can refer to other things pertaining to spiritual elements, or the nature of energy. Much like the word "pneuma" was used by the ancient Greeks to describe the spirit, yet is also the root for "air" in many English words, including the pneumatic (air) pump. Ironically, in Chinese history, according to Zhang Hu Yuan and Ken Rose, in their book "*A Brief History of Qi,*"[6] the word Qi was historically used to describe air, clouds, and the atmosphere. It was not until more modern times that the word Qi became associated with more esoteric aspects.

    The second incidence that further prompted my realization that Qi or oxygen based exercises may be considerably more involved than just blood pumping through the cardiovascular system, came from an article I read in the Los Angeles Times over 15 years ago. The article detailed the use of a "vibrating machine" by researchers at the Rehabilitation Institute of Michigan, which was used to enhance circulation, increase bone density, and reduce muscle spasms.

Feeling the Qi (Oxygen)

"Following a mild stroke, I suffered nerve damage, loss of feeling on my left side, and I had difficulty with my balance. I had been doing therapy and had seen some improvement, but it was not until I tried Tai Chi that something remarkable began to occur. I began to feel a tingling sensation in the fingers of both of my hands, including my left side. The class also helped with my balance and overall physical and mental health."

– Ted. Posted in *"Tai Chi for Health Newsletters."*

Quadriplegics, being bedridden, often suffer from bedsores and poor blood circulation, and need to be turned, massaged, and manipulated on a regular basis (another clue that movement is a necessary requirement for proper blood and oxygen circulation). To prevent the problems associated with being bedridden, the researchers placed the patients on a large platform which would vibrate and shake up the body, similar to a can of paint in a paint mixer at a hardware store.

The idea was that the vibrations would distribute blood and oxygen throughout all of the cells and capillaries in the body, similarly to the way color is distributed throughout a can of paint. And it worked, with some surprising results. Not only did the treatment help eliminate bedsores and poor circulation, but the patients reported what had previously been considered an impossibility – feelings in the extremities of their arms and legs, an indication of nerve re-growth. This study indicated to me that enhanced blood diffusion can result in significant health gains.

The vibrating machine has a parallel in various Chinese health exercises, forms of Qi Gong that involve shaking the body. Many Qi Gong exercises are based on "vibrating" the body through various exercises. As a preliminary to Tai Chi, one common exercise is to vibrate the body through a variety of methods, such as shaking the body up and down very rapidly, or rising up on the toes and then dropping the body so that it "jiggles," or vibrates.

As the body is vibrated, a tingling is felt in the fingers, hands, arms, and sometimes throughout the body, which is seen as enhanced "Qi" flow. This tingling is also felt during Tai Chi and various Qi Gong practices. Thinking on this brought me to the realization that slow movements of the body in exercises such as Tai Chi and Qi Gong may be a health exercise as important in their own right as is aerobics and strength conditioning.

Further supporting the premise that exercises such as Tai Chi enhance oxygen diffusion throughout the entire body, is the incidence of stomach cramps which follow vigorous exercise after a large meal. During vigorous aerobic exercise, the large muscle groups rob the internal organs of oxygen, in order to meet the muscular demands of intense exercise.

Tai Chi Saved My Life

Dr. Roger Jahnke, author of The Healing Promise of Qi *recounted the story of a man with malignant brain cancer. A network of tendrils entwined the brain, and made surgery impossible. Going to China, this person learned and practiced Tai Chi and Qi Gong, in conjunction with herbal and other treatments. A year later, the tumor had shrunk and became benign. Surgeons were able to remove what was left of the tumor.[7]*

So instead of a pleasant tingling as oxygen diffuses throughout the entire body (which occurs during Tai Chi and Qi Gong practice), the body experiences painful cramps as a result of the battle for blood between the stomach and muscles during intense exercise. It should be noted however, that Tai Chi and Qi Gong practitioners also recommend practicing on an empty stomach. Practicing with a full stomach won't result in stomach cramps, but doing these exercises on an empty stomach may optimize blood diffusion throughout the entire body.

Aerobic exercise *is* beneficial in that the circulatory system responds by growing stronger, with an increase in blood vessels, but this does not mean an increase of blood and oxygen, at all levels, or to all areas of the body (particularly at the cellular level within the organs).

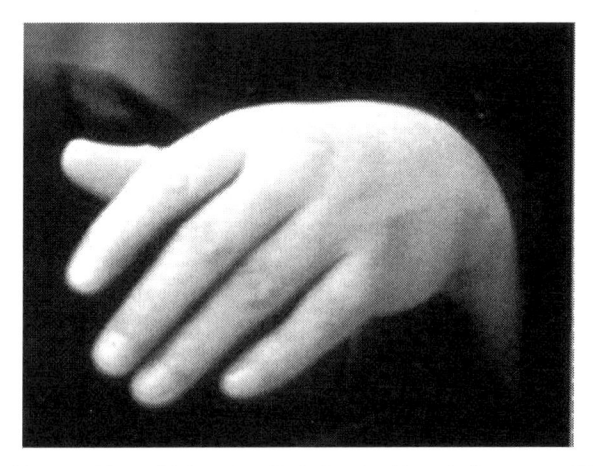

Cheng Man Ching's "Fair Lady Hands" at age 70.
(Photo courtesy of Ken Van Sickle)

Tai Chi and T.B.

In his late twenty's Cheng Man Ching contracted third degree tuberculosis and began coughing up blood. His doctors did not expect him to live beyond 6 months. He began to study Tai Chi diligently and recovered his health, going on to become one of the most well-known Tai Chi teachers of the 20th century.[8]

Based on the tingling feeling in the hands and arms during Tai Chi practice, and in the enhanced blood oxygen saturation as measured with an oximeter, I believe that Metarobic exercises such as Tai Chi and Qi Gong will prove to be particularly effective at enhancing blood oxygen diffusion and metabolic function throughout the entire body, including at the cellular level. Practitioners of forms of Yoga which focus on relaxation and the breath report feeling similar sensations in the body.

The many healing benefits of Tai Chi are supported by a growing body of scientific research, testimonials and news accounts. When I first started Tai Chi practice over 25 years ago, I read an account of an autopsy performed on an older person (I believe the article stated he was 90 or so) who had been a lifetime Tai Chi practitioner. The article stated that the Tai Chi master's organs were more typical of someone in their 30's or 40's. As one ages, a variety of changes occur within the body, including stiffening of the heart, as well as increased arteriosclerosis. The lungs also lose elasticity and the prostate enlarges, while bones can become brittle.[9]

On the previous page is a picture of the hand of Cheng Man Ching when he was 70 year old. In China, Tai Chi is said to preserve youth, reflected in what some Chinese Tai Chi practitioners call "Fair Lady Hands" – soft, supple and firm skin such as is seen in a young woman. The effects of stress and tension is a growing problem in the world, and may also indicate why slow relaxed movements may help increase oxygen flow and thereby health. A common exercise I have beginning students perform is to stand with their hands loose and relaxed at their sides. Most if not all stand with their hands hooked like claws – the result of tension in their lives. One way to gauge the skill level of a Tai Chi practitioner is to look and see how relaxed and "unhooked" their hands are. Tension results in tight muscles, curling the hands into something that looks more like claws than hands. Tense muscles can result in back strain and frozen shoulders or other limbs, in addition to claw like hands. It is not uncommon to see the

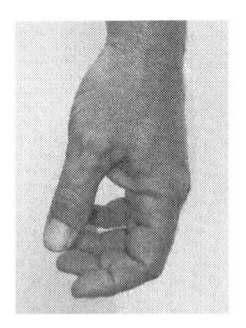

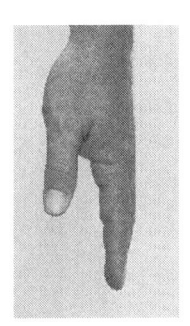

The hand on the left is typical of most people, "clawed" as the result of a life of stress and tension. The hand on the right is more typical of long term Tai Chi practitioners, the result of relaxed muscle tension.

shoulder hunched up in beginning Tai Chi students, or the arm of the "relaxed" arm jutting out to the back due to shoulder and back tension, rather than hanging straight down in a relaxed fashion. Cheng Man Ching, mentioned above, recommended that students visualize the arms and torso as an empty coat hanging from a coat rack, in order to reduce tension in the body. Tension can constrict blood vessels and capillaries, which increases blood pressure and reduces blood flow, and with it the life and energy giving oxygen carried by the blood.

As mentioned earlier, aerobic exercise results in the flow of blood in the body being directed to the large muscle groups that are active, by constricting the capillaries and blood vessels to the organs, and dilating the blood vessels in the large muscle groups. This provides hard working muscles with the oxygen they need. Metarobic theory on the other hand, suggests that by relaxing the muscles, blood flow and oxygen is enhanced to <u>all</u> areas of the body, at what may be a metabolic level.

This does not mean that Metarobics is the best form of exercise, but does indicate that it may be at least as valuable as aerobic and anaerobic exercise for overall health. The heart does not have to work as hard pumping blood through relaxed muscles and an unrestricted vasculature. So what you have is increased blood oxygen saturation and oxygen diffusion due to a relaxed body and deep breathing. Others have also made this inference, as indicated in the case story below.

Tai Chi, Tension, and the Gift of Life

"Bill, a long time Tai Chi practitioner, went in for a complete physical, including a stress test. Fairly shortly into the test, the doctors stopped the test and scheduled an emergency quadruple bypass. Doctors were amazed that Bill had not had a heart attack up to this point – his arteries were 95% occluded. Bill attributed not being short of breath nor experiencing other signs of coronary blockage due to his Tai Chi practice. He felt that the relaxed state of his body permitted maximum blood flow through the blocked arteries. Following the bypass, Bill began a vigorous walking program in conjunction with his Tai Chi, to reap the benefits of both a relaxed body as well as a stronger cardiovascular system."

Personal account related at a Tai Chi practice.

Researchers are capitalizing on the idea of using slow diaphragmatic breathing to train those at risk for high blood pressure, to dilate or open up arteries and reduce blood pressure.[10] Although inspired by meditation practices with a focus on the breath, in this case a device is used to help patients monitor and regulate their breathing. By following tones emitted by the device, the breath is slowed to less than 10 breaths per minute. The end effect is slow deep breathing, enhanced blood flow and reduced blood pressure. A reduction in peripheral resistance (resistance to blood flow due to constricted arteries) and enhanced blood flow was suggested as the mechanism of benefit, as a result of the effects of slow breathing on the sympathetic nervous system.

The sympathetic nervous system helps regulate the body, to activate the body in response to stress – the fight or flight response. Long term activation of the sympathetic nervous system can have negative effects on the body, including increased blood pressure. Slower rates of breathing have been shown to not only reduce blood pressure, but to also result in an increase in arterial oxygen saturation, compared to normal breathing.[11] A focus on Qi, air, the breath – however it is termed – is a key player in health and Metarobic benefits.

Chapter 3

Metarobics and Cancer

The Battle against Hypoxia (Oxygen Deficiency) and the Experiences of Three Students with Cancer

It was the effects of these exercises on three of my students with cancer, which really prompted my curiosity as to how these exercises might be having such dramatic effects on the body. This was the final clue that oxygen use in the body was considerably more critical and comprehensive than just generating chemical energy for the large muscle groups. The first student came to me on the last day of the semester, stating simply that Tai Chi had cured a cancerous lump in her wrist. I am not convinced that the lump in her wrist was cancerous, since cancer is uncommon

Tai Chi Therapy

Tai Chi and Qi Gong Helped Me Battle Lymphoma

Helen Liu had a rare and aggressive form of lymphoma. Chemotherapy failed to eliminate the cancer, and her doctor felt she had only about two weeks left to live. Her father, a famous Kung Fu master (Liang Shou-yu) began Helen on an intensive practice of Qi Gong, Tai Chi, meditation, and alternative forms of Chinese and Western medicine. Helen states: "I was more relaxed, and I was doing Qi Gong and Tai Chi with my dad every day. We'd go out and do all kinds of Qi Gong because it's good for you to stay outside and get a lot of oxygen. That's supposed to kill cancer cells." With all the practices she engaged in, it would be hard to single out Tai Chi and Qi Gong, but for a long time it was a focus of her practice, and is still a regular part of her life 17 years later.

(From Martha Burr, *Kung Fu Tai Chi Magazine*).

---

in this area, but her comments caught me by surprise. After making sure she was seeing her doctor regularly, I thought no more of it.

Two years later another student told me a similar story. He did not want to go into detail, but he said the cancer he had was not responding to chemotherapy, until he started Tai Chi. His cancer disappeared shortly after. Then a year later, during the summer session, a third student who was in the last stages of cancer came to my class. White as a sheet and wearing a bandana to cover her loss of hair, she told me that she had been through all forms of chemo and radiation therapy, but to no avail. Her doctors told her she had about three weeks left to live.

As mentioned in her story at the beginning of this book, Karen was not ready to give up, and decided to try alternative therapies. She had read that Tai Chi can help with cancer, so she came to me. That night I made her a video which talked her through the form. The next day I gave it to her, going over the form with her. Three weeks later, not only was she still alive, but she was completely off of pain pills (she had been taking five maximum doses a day of morphine). Two years later she was still taking the Tai Chi class, before moving to Wyoming to fulfill a lifelong dream. She never experienced complete remission (by the time she began the class, cancer had spread throughout her body), but she had more time to spend with her family, with a better quality of life through her practice of Tai Chi.

At this point I knew there really was a possibility that Tai Chi could have a direct effect on cancer and other conditions. With the first two students, it could have been the radiation and chemotherapy that had made the difference, but the extreme state of this student indicated that Tai Chi (and a Qi Gong exercise called the "Eight Treasures Breathing Exercise," which was also included on the video and in the class) was a major influencing factor.

Following the improvement in Karen's condition, I began researching cancer, and found that there is an extensive body of research related to hypoxia (oxygen deficiency) and cancer. Research into the literature on cancer treatment, described below, indicated that effects on hypoxia and blood oxygen diffusion may be a primary element related to benefits of Tai Chi for cancer and many other conditions.

During this research, I came across the works of Nobel Prize winner Otto Warburg.[1] He found that among the primary types of cancer, affecting over 70% of cancer patients, oxygen restriction seemed to play a critical role. He observed that cancer grew in areas deprived of oxygen, documenting that tumor cells develop a modified sugar based metabolism (glycolysis), rather than oxygen based metabolism, with hypoxic (oxygen deficient) areas surrounding the tumor site. It is not known why cancer cells do this, but current research is offering support that beneficial effects occur from boosting oxygen levels around tumors, which may permit more efficient delivery of chemotherapy and the body's own healing agents.

Part of this research is the work being done at the Birck Nanotechnology Center at Purdue University.[2] Dr. Maleki and colleagues developed a device based on the idea of enhancing tumor oxygenation. The team created an ultrasonically powered micro oxygen generator (IMOG) which can be implanted at the site of the tumor. The IMOG device generates oxygen at the site of the tumor, boosting the cancer fighting power of radiation and chemotherapy. The IMOG device has been used with significant effects in pancreatic tumors in mice, generating oxygen and shrinking tumors faster than without the device.

Tai Chi Was the Best

"A colleague's wife did some Tai Chi and Qi Gong in the final stages of her cancer. She was desperate to try anything that might help. My colleague said that of all the complementary therapies she tried, the one that gave her the most relief from the pain, and helped her anxiety and stress, was Tai Chi."

– David. From *Cancer Active. Tai Chi the Energy Within.*

That enhanced tumor oxygenation resulted in tumor shrinkage, even if only through assisting the effectiveness of radiation and chemotherapy, demonstrates promise for Tai Chi as a cancer preventative and cancer therapy adjunct (keeping in mind to use it in conjunction with prescribed therapies). It is possible that Tai Chi may generate a similar effect to the IMOG device, by increasing blood oxygen saturation and diffusion, and maximizing the body's own natural cancer fighting ability.

Other studies conducted at the University of Texas Anderson Cancer Center noted that the bone marrow microenvironment contains hypoxic areas which inhibit anti-leukemia drugs.[3] Acute lymphoblastic leukemia cells result in marked expansion of hypoxic bone marrow areas, which results in chemoresistance. The authors noted that under conditions of normal oxygen saturation, effectiveness of various forms of chemotherapy was tied to oxygen level, and effectiveness dropped in direct relation to low oxygen levels. Researchers suggest that drugs which target hypoxia may help eliminate leukemia cells within hypoxic areas, and may significantly improve leukemia therapy.

Although Metarobic exercises may not have a target specific effect on lymphoblastic leukemia cells, benefits for cancer care reported in the case stories in this book suggests that these exercises may have a general overall effect on the cancer fighting ability of the body, supported by theoretical elements related to enhanced blood oxygen saturation, diffusion and enhanced oxygen based metabolism. Metarobic exercises may enhance chemo and radiation therapy, at least at a general level (also supported by the uniform reports of benefits for pain management reported by cancer and other patients who practice Tai Chi).

Indeed, it has been further noted that with the central role hypoxia plays in tumor development and resistance to therapy, that tumor hypoxia may be the most valuable and most effective area to target in combating cancer.[4] This suggests that exercises which focus on enhancing oxygen saturation and diffusion throughout the entire body may have at least some effect on combating cancer and other chronic conditions. Needless to say, this would need extensive research to validate and determine exact effects. Of the dozen people in the case stories in this book who reported significant benefits during their cancer treatment, it must be asked, if you had 100 patients with the same form of cancer, who all practiced specific user friendly forms of Tai Chi, Qi Gong or other Metarobic exercises, what percentage would benefit and to what degree?

The Amazing Results of Qi Gong

"Five years ago, I was found to have cancer. I had a tumor on my larynx and throughout the five weeks of super-voltage radiation, I practiced The Eight Precious Sets of Exercises known to the Chinese as Ba Duan Jin. This was not only a great source of physical and mental wellbeing, but it produced tangible and somewhat amazing results. Exposure to intense radiation is expected to have its negative side effects...weight loss, loss of appetite, loss of sleep and a general downturn in spirit are the most typical. I am glad to say that at no time did I experience any of these. Even case hardened doctors and nurses were impressed and asked me to demonstrate the Precious Set of Eight. Today at 50 I am fit, healthy and a great believer in these exercises. I have no way of proving how much their daily practice had to do with my recovery, but I do know that they have given me a new outlook and renewed vitality."

– Geoff Pike (From *"The Power of Qi"*).

The literature on cancer research abounds with studies related to the effects, impact, or implications of hypoxia (oxygen deficiency) and cancer. Research has documented that tumors result in hypoxic areas, due to growth distancing tumor cells from the surrounding capillaries.[5,6] Solid tumors often have large areas of acute and chronic hypoxia, which is associated with aggressive tumor expansion and poor outcomes for radiotherapy and chemotherapy. Reoxygenation is an important aspect of tumor therapy and positive response to therapy.[5] Metarobic theory suggests that enhanced blood diffusion may decrease levels of hypoxia around tumor sites, and increase oxygen levels in hypoxic areas.

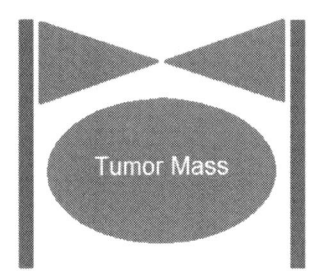

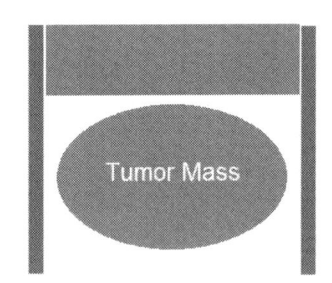

Illustration of hypoxic tumor mass (adapted from "Hypoxia and Cancer" by Brahimi-Horn and colleagues), and possible effects of Tai Chi and IMOG device.

As mentioned earlier, it is common when performing Tai Chi to feel a pleasant tingling in the hands and arms, indicating increased oxygen diffusion. By enhancing blood oxygen saturation and diffusion, it may be possible to boost oxygen delivery to hypoxic areas. One drug which is affected by hypoxia is salicylic acid (the active ingredient in aspirin). Salicylic acid is noted to reduce risk of colon cancer. But salicylic acid has been found to be non-effective under hypoxic conditions.[7] In the study, the effects of salicylic acid on colon cancer cells was found to be dependent on the availability of oxygen. Greater hypoxia is directly related to the stage of cancer and treatment resistance.

Remarkable Progress Through Qi Gong

"I have gone through 16 chemotherapy treatments and 20 sessions of radiation. I also had 22 blood transfusions in about 5 months. The medical doctors did not know what to do with me. After doing Qi Gong, my bleeding has completely stopped after eleven weeks, which is a miracle. The doctors had given up and referred me to end of life care, and they expected me to die. A CAT scan taken five months later shows remarkable progress. I have not let a day go by without practicing my Qi Gong."

- Cristela Gutierrez
(From *The Seventh Happiness School of Chi Gong*)

Dyspnea, or shortness of breath, is common in patients with cancer.[8] The cause of dyspnea in cancer patients is not currently known. Patients with cancer were found to have reduced diffusing capacity of the lungs for carbon monoxide, and reduced skeletal muscle strength, resulting in shortness of breath, as the body struggles to bring in more oxygen. Researchers suggest that muscle weakness in the chest and diaphragm may be one possible explanation for increased shortness of breath. Tai Chi and similar metarobic exercises may provide a method to reduce shortness of breath, either through enhancing the diffusing capacity of the lungs, or by increasing skeletal muscle strength and capacity through the deep breathing aspect, or possibly in combination.

Researchers have also noted that intermittent hypoxia can promote cancer tumor growth.[9] In a study of 1,522 people with sleep-disordered breathing (such as sleep apnea), repeated hypoxemia (low oxygen) was found to be associated with profound metabolic disruption. Even with adjustments for age, sex, body mass and smoking, sleep-disordered breathing resulted in a significant increase in cancer deaths of up to 4.8 times the number of deaths from cancer in the normal population.

Another indication that oxygen levels in the body may directly affect cancer development is the rare occurrence of cancer in red muscle tissue. Cancer rarely occurs in striated muscles (the large muscle groups that connect the skeleton, such as the leg and arm muscles).[10] This may be due to the oxygen rich environment of skeletal muscles. As observed from stomach cramps that occur when exercising strenuously after a full meal, the major muscle groups have the ability to command the oxygen supply and blood flow in the body during exercise.

Tai chi and similar Metarobic exercises may have the benefit of enhancing blood flow to *all* areas of the body. Such exercises may provide a means to boost cellular health and functioning throughout the body, in ways unique from conventional exercises, impacting a wide range of health conditions, including cancer prevention and treatment. And although the vote may be out in the medical community regarding a direct effect on cancer, as a whole, Tai Chi and similar Metarobic exercises have been found to reduce negative side effects of cancer treatment, and provide a low impact method of enhancing health.

STUDIES ON TAI CHI AND CANCER

In a recent review of 13 randomized controlled trails investigating the benefits of Tai Chi and Qi Gong as an adjunct to cancer care, positive effects were found for cancer specific improved quality of life, reduction of fatigue, enhanced immune function, and reduced cortisol levels.[11] Cortisol acts to increase blood sugar by gluconeogenesis, and also suppresses the immune system and can decrease bone formation. Researchers at the Wilmot Cancer Center at University of Rochester in New York, suggest direct effects on the regulation of inflammatory responses related to cancer treatment, and effects on overall quality of life during cancer care and treatment.[12]

Tai Chi Gives Me The Strength To Deal With Cancer

"Tai Chi really gives my body strength to put up with the pains of my breast cancer and back problems. Tai Chi is 'sneaky'. You don't think it's helping, but eventually you realize it's helping you."

Unknown. From *Faulk Tai Chi*.

A systematic inflammatory response has been observed to be associated with consistently worse outcomes in early and late stage cancers.[13] Aside from anti-inflammatory effects of Tai Chi, benefits have also been reported for bone density. Tai Chi can also have an effect on antioxidant capacity, which can affect cancer development. Following eight weeks of Tai Chi classes four times a week, participants in another study experienced an increase in aerobic responsive antioxidant enzymes and plasma total antioxidant status.[14] Antioxidants are important for fighting oxidative stress related metabolic diseases, which can result in toxic effects damaging all components of a cell, including proteins, lipids and DNA.

Oxidative stress is considered a primary factor in the development of cancer, as well as in Parkinson's disease, Alzheimer's, heart disease, and many other conditions. Oxidative stress is the result of activated oxygen molecules (reactive oxygen) which can cause cell damage. In short, and in plain English, oxygen based metabolism results in harmful byproducts, much like burning gasoline in a car results in harmful pollution to the environment. Tai Chi and other Metarobic exercise, based on these and other studies, may reduce or reverses oxidative stress, by enhancing the process of oxygen based metabolism, reducing harmful byproducts.

Current studies strongly indicate that Tai Chi and related exercises enhance metabolic processes. This would account at least in part for many of the benefits of Metarobic based exercises. By enhancing efficient use of oxygen throughout the entire body, Metarobic exercises may impact everything from the metabolic process, to the manufacture of proteins and other molecules (as noted in the study by Dr. Kuender Yang[15] in Chapter Six: *Metarobics for Immunity, Diabetes, and Pain*). Metarobic exercises, from Tai Chi to forms of Yoga and Qi Gong, and new exercises yet to come, may be a major missing link for total health and disease prevention.

Not a Hair Lost during Chemo Thanks to Yoga

My Yoga teacher told me of a woman with brain cancer who had undergone surgery, but had then been given three months to live. She then began Yoga with him. He said it was four years since she has been cured. So I had my mother do Yoga, since she had been diagnosed with stage three cancer of the uterus. Doctors had given my mother a 25-30 percent chances of survival. She did chemotherapy and radiotheraphy sessions simultaneously with the Yoga therapy, which included a diet regimen. My mother is doing absolutely fine now. She did not lose even a strand of hair despite intensive chemotherapy.

– Bhavna (From *The Health Site*)

CONCLUSION

From the roots of Qi as "air," to my experiences with three students with cancer and a growing body of research, it became obvious that there are measureable mechanisms related to oxygen behind many if not all of the benefits of Tai Chi and various forms of Qi Gong and Yoga for health. Physiological mechanisms for benefits do not necessarily discount elements related to energy work, or metaphysical and mystical elements, for those who are fascinated by the range and depth of these exercises (see the conclusion at the end of this book for a discussion of the more esoteric elements of these exercises). Indeed, even exercises such as running have been attributed with spiritual aspects, not to mention the runners' high.[16]

Use the material in this book to enhance your health, if your find it meaningful to your condition. But the reader is cautioned to keep their doctors advice in mind as well. If using any of these exercises for a medical condition, use them in conjunction with your doctors' recommendations, and in consultation with your doctor. Tai Chi classes, styles and teaching methodology can vary considerably as well, elaborated on in Chapter Seven: *Essential Elements of Metarobics and Tai Chi for Therapy*.

Doctors Call Me a "Walking Miracle"

"Conventional cancer treatment didn't work the first time. I was resolved to find alternative measures to find healing. After six, seven months of both medical treatments and Qigong I am completely healed. My cancer's gone. My doctors call me a 'walking miracle'."

– Karyn (From *Spring Forest Qi Gong Testimonials*)

Chapter 4

Metarobics, Heart Disease, Stroke and Kidney Disease

Dealing with the Pressure of Life

Cardiovascular disease, also known as heart disease, is strongly linked to diet and inactivity, and is the number one cause of death in the United States. Plaque buildup in the arteries which supply blood to the heart is called coronary artery disease. Plaque build-up is generally the result of a diet high in saturated fats. The plaque literally "clogs" the arteries so that blood cannot get to the heart in sufficient quantity, much like a clog of hair creates a slow moving drain. Atherosclerosis, or hardening of the arteries, is also caused by a buildup of plaque.

Restricted blood flow to the organs can result in hardening of the arteries due to increased pressure on the arteries. Heart attacks can result from heart disease, when blood clots and is prevented from reaching the heart. According to an American Hospital Association report, currently one in three American adults have some form of cardiovascular disease.[1] The Center for Disease Control (CDC) states that heart disease accounts for almost 700,000 deaths each year.[2] It is also almost entirely preventable.

Tai Chi Prevented a Heart Attack

Maggie told me that she had been a long time Tai Chi practitioner, but did not do other exercises. She went in for a stress test, and the doctors were surprised to find her arteries were over 90 percent blocked. Maggie was rushed in for a bypass, but following the operation, she stated that her heart would not resume a regular heartbeat. She was told that she would need a pacemaker. The doctors were about to send her back into the operating room. But for some reason, Maggie felt that if she could just do Tai Chi, that her heart would be okay. She asked to be left alone for an hour, did Tai Chi, and when the doctors came back, her heart had stabilized. The doctors were surprised, and told her "whatever you are doing, keep doing it." Maggie stated: "The moral of the story is that even with Tai Chi, a good diet and cardio exercise are still necessary, but Tai Chi did keep me going until I got the bypass, and got my heart back to beating normally. So now I do both (cardio and Tai Chi)."

Personal Story Related at a Tai Chi Workshop.

The key element in relation to Metarobic theory is restricted blood flow to various areas of the body, in this case the heart or brain, which can also increase blood pressure. Metarobic exercises such as Tai Chi relax muscle tension in the body, and has a direct effect on blood pressure, documented in numerous studies (highlighted below). It may also be possible that enhanced metabolic function via Tai Chi may even affect cholesterol metabolism. More efficient cholesterol metabolism may help moderate the balance of HDL cholesterol (which carries away deposits), and LDL cholesterol (which leaves deposits and can lead to a heart attack or stroke). Hypoxia can underlie problems with managing cholesterol. According to a study conducted at John Hopkins University, intermittent hypoxia is associated with hypercholesterolemia (extreme levels of cholesterol in the blood), as a result of obstructive sleep apnea, which can occur as a result of intermittent or partial blockage of the airways during sleep.[3]

Beneficial effects of Tai Chi on blood pressure is related to the slow pace with the focus on relaxation. Blood pressure is the force or pressure of blood inside the arteries. If you did not have any blood pressure, the pumping of the heart would have little effect on moving blood throughout the body. It would be like the anemic trickle of water that comes from a shower which has low water pressure. Higher water pressure means more water moving through the pipes. Too much water pressure and the pipes could burst. The same is true for blood vessels, as well as for the heart – too much pressure in the heart, and it becomes enlarged and pumping efficiency is reduced.

Tai Chi Lowered My Chronic High Blood Pressure

"I had chronic high blood pressure, and suffered from tense neck and shoulder muscles from the stress at work. I was on the verge of burnout and at risk for cardiovascular disease, when I started Tai Chi. Since learning Tai Chi, my blood pressure is back to normal, and I have a feeling of peacefulness and well-being that I carry into my work and family life. I would recommend Tai Chi to everyone – you have nothing to lose and so much to gain!"

– Natalie (Posted On: *Tai Chi for Life Online Magazine*).

The dynamic state of relaxation generated from Tai Chi and similar metarobic exercises may relax not just the large muscle groups, but also the arteries. Researchers at the University of North Texas noted a relationship between flexibility as determined by the sit and reach test (sitting on the floor and seeing how far you can reach towards your toes) and arterial health.[4] Supple arterial walls require the heart to work less to pump blood throughout the body, while stiff arteries require the heart to work harder, and can contribute to a greater risk for heart attack and stroke. The researchers found a significant relationship between flexibility and arterial stiffness – the stiffer and less flexible the participants were, the higher the readings they had in arterial stiffness.

Before I started Tai Chi, I could barely reach past my knees in the sit and reach test. After several years of Tai Chi and Qi Gong, my flexibility increased to where I could bend over and place the palms of my hands flat on the floor. This was before I began any kind of stretching regimen. As I got older I realized the importance of stretching, particularly after exercising, so I now also stretch after vigorous exercise. However, although Tai Chi and related exercises may result in more efficient blood flow, and possibly even greater arterial flexibility, there is no evidence to date that it can reverse or prevent plaque build-up.

Ultimately, it may be important to develop a multifaceted exercise program, one involving aerobic, anaerobic *and* Metarobic exercise, as well as stretching. Although Tai Chi is not classified as a vigorous exercise, the relaxation and breath aspects are a valuable addition to an aerobic program, as highlighted throughout this book. In my own practice, I also engage in various forms of cardiovascular exercise and strength training, using exercises based on traditional Kung Fu aimed at the total health of the mind and body. Working to enhance health from a Metarobic, aerobic and anaerobic perspective.

Metarobic exercises are important for the relaxation aspect, for promoting an unrestricted pliable vasculature and lowering blood pressure, which research supports as helping to prevent heart attacks, stroke and kidney disease. Although we tend to think of muscle tension as affecting just the large muscle groups, arteries are composed of sheaths of smooth muscles, which can also be affected by muscle tension. Even mental tension, in the form of various stressors, can result in constriction of blood vessels, raising blood pressure.[5]

Tai Chi Controls My Blood Pressure

"My Blood Pressure was edging towards an unhealthy high, but I did not want to take drugs. I was fortunate in that my doctor supported trying Tai Chi first. As I continued with Tai Chi my blood pressure gradually dropped. After several months, my blood pressure had dropped from 150/90 mmHg to 134/82. Every time I do Tai Chi I feel so much better. I have even learned to control my blood pressure when I get stressed. When I begin to feel stressed, I can practice Tai Chi's open-close breathing, and it lowers my blood pressure almost immediately.

– Marilyn (Posted On: *Heart Healthy Living*).

Calcium-channel blockers are prescribed for people with high blood pressure to chemically reduce muscle tension in arteries, as well as to relax blood vessels, to create a greater capacity for blood flow. These drugs also slightly relax the heart muscle, resulting in a slower heartbeat, which also reduces blood pressure. Calcium-channel blockers are used to control blood pressure to help prevent strokes, heart attacks and kidney disease. But like many medications, calcium channel blockers also carry a risk, sometimes fatal.[6]

Tai Chi practice and the theories involved in Metarobics are new enough that exact mechanisms have not been scientifically verified. But it is worth investigating if the dynamic state of physical relaxation extends not just to the large muscle groups, but also to tension in all of the muscles of the body, including the artery walls and heart. A mechanism related to the relaxation component of Tai Chi seems probable from an intuitive perspective, and is worth future research to determine the exact mechanisms. The end of this chapter details studies on the benefits of Metarobics exercises on blood pressure and relevant conditions.

Strokes and Tai Chi

Strokes can also result from cardiovascular disease, and are the third leading cause of death, following cancer. A stroke can be considered a "brain attack," the blocking of an artery to the brain by a blood clot, or the rupturing of a blood vessel in the brain. According to the National Stroke Association, 80 percent of strokes are preventable.[7] Strokes and heart attacks can both result from high blood pressure, which is considered one of the most important modifiable risk factors.

Tai Chi Helped Me Recover My Life After A Stroke

"Four years ago I had a minor stroke which affected my left side. I experienced weakness, loss of balance, and I was inclined to throw my left foot when walking. After three weeks of therapy at a local hospital there was some improvement, but I was very stressed about it. Then my doctor suggested I try Tai Chi. I attended that class for two years. I am happy to say that my balance has improved 80%, my strength 70%, and I no longer throw my left foot. I can once again enjoy long walks."

– James. (Posted On: *Tai Chi Fitness for Health*).

Smoking and alcohol use, as well as being overweight, can increase your risk for stroke, as well as for heart attacks and kidney disease. Surprisingly, Tai Chi may also help to control addiction to smoking, alcohol and other substances as a form of mindfulness based meditation. Mindfulness based practices have been used to target addiction to destructive behaviors for over a millennia. Research indicates mindfulness based practices have applications for physical addictions as well, which is discussed in the conclusion of this book.

Returning to increased risk factors for stroke, people with high cholesterol can experience higher blood pressure during stressful situations than those with lower levels of cholesterol.[8] This also supports the benefits of exercises such as Tai Chi, as a meditative exercises for dealing with stress, as well as for relaxing muscle tension. As noted earlier, research indicates that high cholesterol may reduce the ability of blood vessels to relax and constrict normally, since blood vessel constriction results in an increase of blood pressure.[8]

Tai Chi has been demonstrated in numerous studies to be effective in lowering blood pressure. If you are at particular risk due to genetics or lifestyle, enhanced blood diffusion and blood oxygen saturation may help delay incidence of stroke or heart attack, until it is detected by your physician (as indicated by the case story on the following page). If you are of healthy weight and engaged in a regular cardiovascular program, Tai Chi may help maximize blood diffusion and oxygen saturation, to maximize the benefits of aerobic exercise, as well as to help maintain healthy blood pressure. Tai Chi may also help maintain or restore a normal heartbeat, as noted by the case story of Maggie presented at the beginning of this chapter. Atrial fibrillation is an abnormal heartbeat which can increase the risk of stroke by 500 percent, causing blood to pool in the heart, which may form a clot and result in a stroke.

Although approximately 87 percent of strokes result from blocked arteries as a result of blood clots or buildup of plaque and other fatty deposits (called ischemic strokes),[9] blood vessels in the brain can rupture due to weak spots in the walls of blood vessels, resulting in hemorrhagic strokes.[10]

Tai Chi, Tension, and the Gift of Life

"Bill, a long time Tai Chi practitioner, went in for a complete physical, including a stress test. Fairly shortly into the test, the doctors stopped the test and scheduled an emergency quadruple bypass. Doctors were amazed that Bill had not had a heart attack up to this point – his arteries were 95% occluded. Bill attributed not being short of breath nor experiencing other signs of coronary blockage due to his Tai Chi practice. He felt that the relaxed state of his body permitted maximum blood flow through the blocked arteries. Following the bypass, Bill began a vigorous walking program in conjunction with his Tai Chi, to reap the benefits of both a relaxed body as well as a stronger cardiovascular system."

Personal account related at a Tai Chi practice.

Some Qi Gong (breathing exercises) may act in other ways to reduce the risk of stroke as well, by momentarily increasing blood pressure to strengthen artery walls (which would need to be confirmed with research). Pa Duan Jin, the "eight treasures" or "eight pieces of silk brocade" exercise, may strengthen blood vessel walls in healthy adults as a result of brief momentary spikes in blood pressure, during those poses which are preformed inverted, or while holding the breath. During the movement "press the earth, touch the sky," the hands touch the toes (or as low as you can reach). When you bend over, the blood pressure in the head spikes momentarily (the body is well designed to respond quickly to changes in body position). This movement may help strengthen the blood vessels of the brain, again by momentarily stressing them, so that they respond by growing stronger.

There are also two poses performed with a momentary holding of the breath, which may increase internal pressure during the range of movement. Needless to say, scientific studies would need to be conducted to verify the exact benefits of these poses. But from a theoretical viewpoint, increasing internal pressure for brief moments may benefit not only the strength of blood vessel walls, but may also enhance diffusion of life giving blood and the elements it carries, by enhancing osmosis through the cells of the body (including oxygen molecules).

Needless to say, inverted poses may not be beneficial for those who have uncontrolled high blood pressure, or with other risk factors for stroke, and stresses the importance of discussing any new health routine with your doctor. The same may be true for those poses in which the body is momentarily "pressurized," by holding the breath while going through a pose. These movements, performed for only a few seconds, may provide benefits for healthy adults, but should be discussed with your doctor if you are in doubt. Those with uncontrolled high blood pressure or other conditions may be advised to avoid anything which may affect blood pressure upward, even if only momentarily.

It should be noted that some forms of martial arts Qi Gong use unorthodox forms of breathing for prolonged periods to "pressurize" the body, to make it more resistant to blows. These forms of breathing may actually cause dangerous increases in blood pressure, and over time may lead to severe health problems, including heart failure. In ancient times, when a person's life depended on surviving various battles, such a practice might be worth the tradeoff for a shorter life expectancy, but for modern practice it is generally better to stay away from more esoteric forms of breathing.

Diaphragmatic or abdominal breathing, has been shown to be safe and effective, and a much healthier way of breathing than shallow chest breathing. For most Qi Gong exercises this is the best form to use. More details on breathing for Tai Chi and Qi Gong are given in Chapter Seven: *Essential Elements of Metarobics and Tai Chi for Therapy*.

Tai Chi and Kidney Disease

High blood pressure is also a major risk factor for kidney disease, which is another leading cause of early death in the United States. Kidney disease, also known as renal disease, is the result of conditions which can damage the kidneys. Damaged kidneys can result in the build-up of wastes in your blood, which can result in a wide range of health concerns. Kidney disease can be caused by a variety of conditions, including high blood pressure, which puts one at higher risk for this disease. Diabetes can also cause kidney disease.

Tai Chi Saved My Life From Kidney Disease

"Luo Ji Hong got kidney disease sometime in his 30's and ended up needing surgery, during which his left kidney was removed. It was also discovered that his right kidney was deteriorating as well. The doctors said there was nothing they could do. Luo's kidney was failing, and he was given five months left to live. A friend suggested he try Tai Chi. Lou decided to try it, and from then on he left the hospital every morning to practice Tai Chi at a local school. Lou and the doctors were amazed, when he began to feel better after just a month of practice. After an examination, the doctor found that his remaining kidney has stopped deteriorating. The internal bleeding had also stopped. Six months later Luo was back to a healthy weight, to the amazement of his doctors. Thirty years later he was still practicing Tai Chi, knowing it had saved his life."

– Luo Ji Hong
(Posted On: *Luo Ji-Hong. A Life Through Tai Chi*).

According to the American Heart Association, high blood pressure can seriously affect kidneys due to the dense supply of blood vessels in the kidneys and the high volume of blood flow.[11] High blood pressure can damage the arteries around the kidneys, resulting in insufficient blood flow to the kidneys. Kidneys filter blood through small finger like nephrons. Damaged arteries result in a reduction of blood flow, the ability to filter blood, and impacts the supply of essential oxygen and nutrients to the kidneys.

It is interesting to note that hypoxia and lack of oxygen is also mentioned in the various studies related to the development of kidney disease reviewed below. Since Metarobics is new as a theory of health and exercise, a good deal of scientific testing needs to be conducted to verify and document exactly how Metarobic based exercises may affect kidney and other diseases, but the trend and observations indicate an important area for future research. As for the relaxation factor in reducing blood pressure and possible effects on kidney disease, it is worth noting that the American Heart Association states that managing blood pressure is an important part of prolonging kidney health.[11]

Kidney hypoxia has a pivotal role in the development and outcome of acute and chronic kidney disease, according to a growing body of research.[12-16] Chronic hypoxia has been identified as a probable central mechanism and final pathway to chronic kidney disease involving a loss of renal function. When local metabolism is disturbed by an imbalance between oxygen supply and consumption, hypoxia can result.[12]

Researchers have observed that the body can respond to hypoxia through a protein called hypoxia-inducible factor, which can help the body to fight hypoxia by causing cells to regress to a less differentiated cell type.[13] However, hypoxia inducible factor is also implicated in cancer under negative conditions, and overall can result in the synthesis of fibrous tissues interfering with the kidneys normal filtering functions. Considering that a discrepancy between oxygen demand and availability is common to most chronic kidney diseases,[13] Metarobic exercises may enhance positive conditions. Evidence suggests that this may be a result of negating activation of a hypoxia inducible factor, and the restoration of oxygen supply, resulting in the support of healthy metabolic function.

The kidney is particularly sensitive to oxygen delivery,[14] supporting the premise that benefits for kidney disease resulting from exercises such as Tai Chi may be due to enhanced oxygen delivery and diffusion. Since kidney hypoxia has a pivotal role in the development and outcome of acute and chronic kidney disease, hypoxia has been targeted as a prime target for therapeutic interventions.[12-15] Hypoxia can also result in inflammation with the progression of kidney disease, since hypoxia signals injury to the body. This signal results in an increase of immune cells, leading to inflammation.[15] Therapies targeting hypoxia have the potential to reduce the progression of kidney disease. Tai Chi Therapy may be one viable option.

Even more relevant to the theory of Metarobics is a study conducted at Lariboisiere Hospital in Paris.[16] Researchers noted that micro-vascular dysfunction may result from an imbalance between a variety of factors (such as mitochondrial dysfunction and activity of alternative oxygen consuming pathways). This can lead to decreased kidney oxygen supply. It was noted that a reduction in micro-circulatory oxygen supply may contribute to kidney dysfunction. Kidneys have less oxygen reserves than other organs, and are even more susceptible to reduced capillary blood flow. Future studies on the effects of Metarobic exercises on capillary blood flow and kidney oxygen supply may yield some promising effects, as a means to enhance blood flow throughout the muscles *and* the organs.

Scientific Studies on the Effects of Tai Chi on Blood Pressure, Heart Disease and Stroke

The effect of Tai Chi on blood pressure is one of the most studied areas in Tai Chi research. Dr. Gloria Yeh, a researcher at Harvard Medical School, along with three colleagues, conducted an extensive review of studies examining the effects of Tai Chi on cardiovascular disease, associated risk factors, and blood pressure.[17,18]

Clear Speech and New Feeling through Tai Chi

"I started Tai Chi because of my stroke. My body is different now, and not only has it helped me with balance, my friends have noticed improvements too! My speech has become clearer and my step is more sure-footed. I can navigate steps that once intimidated me. I am also noticing new feelings in my left arm and leg."

– Bob (From: *Tai Chi Chih. What Others Are Saying*).

One study reviewed consisted of an eight week program for patients recovering from an acute heart attack (myocardial infarction). This program resulted in a significant reduction in systolic and diastolic blood pressure in the Tai Chi group. Participants were randomly assigned to either the Tai Chi group or to an aerobic exercise group. The aerobic group exhibited a decrease in systolic blood pressure, but not in diastolic blood pressure. Tai Chi reduced both factors. The Tai Chi group also experienced a decrease in resting heart rate. Participants in this group also had greater attendance in the Tai Chi class, compared to the aerobic exercise group.

Two studies in Dr. Yeh's review examined the effect of Tai Chi on heart failure. Tai chi resulted in a significant increase in exercise capacity, as measured by a six minute walk test. Participants also experienced improved disease specific quality of life, and had a significant reduction in a polypeptide (BNP), which when high is an indicator of excessive stretching of heart muscle cells. In another study comparing Tai Chi, moderate-intensity walking, and low-impact aerobics, all three groups experienced a similar reduction in blood pressure. The Tai Chi group also had the highest exercise compliance (attendance and regular practice) in this study as well.

Regular exercise has long been advocated as a way to reduce or prevent high blood pressure, and Metarobic based exercises provide one more option. Dr. Yeh also noted a study which reported significant reductions compared to normal hospital care in total cholesterol, low-density lipoprotein, and triglycerides, using a twelve week Tai Chi program for patients with hypertension. Overall, it was suggested that Tai Chi may be particularly valuable for those who cannot participate in more vigorous forms of exercise.

Studies conducted since Dr. Yeh's reviews continue to support the benefits of Tai Chi for lowering blood pressure. Tai Chi has been shown to have a direct effect on baroreflex sensitivity in those with coronary heart disease.[19] The baroreflex is a physical mechanism for maintaining blood pressure. High blood pressure triggers a decrease in heart rate, which results in lowered blood pressure. In a comparison of conventional cardiac rehabilitation program to a program which also included Tai Chi, the conventional care group showed no significant changes in baroreflex sensitivity, while those in the Tai Chi group demonstrated statistically significant improvement.

High blood pressure is such a concern for cardiovascular health, that it is one of the most studied areas, yielding a number of reviews. An extensive review conducted in 2012 further supported benefits from Tai Chi, which included a significant increase in quality of life, as measured by the Minnesota Living with Heart Failure Questionnaire (MLHFQ), as well as a decrease in polypeptide (BNP, which as mentioned above, is an indicator of excessive stretching of heart muscle cells, and is a marker used to diagnose heart failure).[20]

Benefits were also reported for better sleep quality, improvement in left ventricular ejection fraction (a measurement of how much blood is pumped out of the main chamber of the heart), and a significant improvement in peak rate pressure product (PRPP – an indirect measure of myocardial work) compared to standard care, as well as an increase in peak oxygen uptake and exercise intensity (compared to a slight decrease in a walk group).

The reviewers concluded that Tai Chi may improve cardiac function, modify risk factors, enhance quality of life, improve heart rate, heart rate response, blood pressure, baroreflex sensitivity, blood volume ejection, peak oxygen uptake, and exercise intensity.[20] Overall, Tai Chi practice improved a large variety of factors important for controlling or preventing high blood pressure. It is also important to note that no adverse effects were reported, unlike some forms of blood pressure medication, which can result in a variety of unintended effects, including death if taking too high doses of medication (again indicating the importance of following any regimen closely with your doctor).

Another study conducted at the University of Liverpool compared an older adult group of sedentary women to a comparable group enrolled in a Tai Chi class.[21] The women in the Tai Chi group experienced significant improvements not just in blood pressure, but also in balance (death and injury from falls is a major risk factor in older adults). The Tai Chi group experienced an average decrease in systolic pressure of 9.71, and an average decrease in diastolic pressure of 7.53.

From a Metarobic perspective, it is particularly worth noting the increase in peak oxygen uptake. In this case, researchers believe the mechanism of action may be related to the improvement of microcirculatory function. One of the basic premises of Metarobics is that it positively affects microcirculation and enhances blood diffusion. It is also important to not overlook the mind/body connection of these exercises, particularly related to stress. Research suggests that Tai Chi has an effect on the physiological stress management mechanisms as well (discussed in the conclusion of this book).

Tai Chi has also been used successfully for survivors of stroke, in order to enhance balance, quality of life, and mental health.[22] Chapter Seven: *Essential Elements of Metarobics and Tai Chi Therapy*, presents the structural and practical aspects of Tai Chi which enhance balance.

The Medical World Needs To Know About Tai Chi

"Following a stroke, I was unable to walk more than 50 feet or so, and ended up confined to a wheelchair. I heard about a program for wheelchair Tai Chi, and began going twice a week. Two months later I could walk and even climb stairs without help, and got back some use of my left arm. I feel like I have accomplished something, and it's easy and fun. The medical world should be aware that people need something like this."

– Mrs. B. (From *Kungfumagazine.com. Tai Chi as Medicine*).

From a Metarobic perspective, Tai Chi may also affect heart disease by bringing in extra oxygen through the deep breathing aspect and through enhanced blood flow and microcirculation, by creating a relaxed body and unrestricted vasculature (as indicated by the case stories presented in this chapter). Preliminary evidence suggests that Tai Chi may result in more efficient function of the autonomic nervous system and overall physiological function of the body and relevant hormones, to moderate blood pressure through a variety of mechanisms.

As a low impact exercise, the above research supports that Tai Chi and related exercises are a particularly valuable adjunct for cardiac rehabilitation, under a physician's supervision, and in conjunction with conventional care.

Other Considerations

Although Tai Chi aids in relaxing muscle tension and directly impacts blood pressure, it is not vigorous enough to have the same benefits for cardiovascular health that aerobic exercise does. A complete health regimen may need to incorporate all elements of fitness, including diet, aerobic exercise, anaerobic exercise and stretching, as well as Metarobics. Tai Chi does have the potential to fulfill all of these categories, including an impact on diet through the development of mindfulness (discussed in the conclusion). By also performing Tai Chi at full speed (in addition to regular slow practice), similar to Kung Fu and Karate forms, the heart rate can be elevated to aerobic levels.

The traditional 108 Yang long form, which traditionally takes between 20-40 minutes to perform when done slowly, can also be completed in under two minutes when done at full speed. This results in a fast paced aerobic exercise that can get you as out of breath as any cycling class. Of course it would mean 10 to 20 repetitions of the form to get your 30 minutes of exercise. An alternative for aerobic conditioning is to repeat individual movements at a fast pace, similar to the way Billy Blanks adapted kickboxing in his popular Tae Bo exercises. I have used this method in college classes with great success, to demonstrate the versatility of Tai Chi. Traditional martial training of Tai Chi includes a 'fast set' of Tai Chi.

The need for some basic form of strength training, valuable for enhancing functionality into old age, can be achieved by using wrist or hand weights, to increase muscle tone in the upper body (the knees and legs are strengthened through the bent knees and lowered stance used when performing Tai Chi). Incorporating Tai Chi weapon sets can also add an element of strength training, as well as aerobic exercise, when the weapon sets are performed at higher speeds (traditional forms of Tai Chi, originating as a martial art, also included various weapons practice, such as the straight sword and broadsword). Systematically rotating the way you practice Tai Chi can address cardiovascular and strength benefits, as well as Metarobic benefits from slow relaxed practice.

Chapter 5

Metarobics, Lung Disease and Asthma

Better Breathing through Tai Chi and Qi Gong

Metarobic exercises such as Tai Chi and various forms of Qi Gong, having been developed to maximize efficient use of oxygen and respiration, can have positive effects on the many conditions associated with forms of chronic respiratory diseases. Chronic lower respiratory disease is the third leading cause of death in the United States. It can result from a variety of factors and is an umbrella term for a variety of conditions. Essentially chronic respiratory disease can be seen as an ongoing difficulty with breathing. The two primary forms of chronic respiratory disease are asthma and chronic obstructive pulmonary disease (COPD).[1,2]

The Center for Disease Control states that approximately 25 million people in the United States have asthma, or about one out of every twelve people, and that this number is growing every year.[2] Another 13.1 million Americans have been diagnosed with chronic obstructive pulmonary disease (COPD), with 24 million more adults living with impaired lung function, which is an indication and precursor of COPD.[1]

Tai Chi Helped My Asthma, And Cured My Back Pain Too!

"I developed asthma more than 20 years ago. For the last 15 years, I have had to use an inhaler several times a day. After starting Tai Chi, my posture improved and in 7 – 8 months there was dramatic improvement. I no longer feared not having my inhaler with me, and over time stopped carrying it. As I write this, I realize that except for one setback, I have not had an episode in two to three months. And my back pain has disappeared too."

– Kenneth G. (Posted On: *ChiArts.com*).

* Note: Despite the affirmation of how Tai Chi helped his asthma, it is not recommended to discontinue carrying an inhaler, unless approved by your doctor.

COPD is an umbrella term for two lung diseases, emphysema and chronic bronchitis, characterized by obstruction to airflow which interferes with normal breathing.[1] This chapter will also look at the promising elements of Metarobic exercises for asthma as well, since asthma shares some elements in common with COPD (as a chronic long term respiratory disease, which inflames and narrows the airways, and interferes with breathing).

Cigarette smoking is the primary risk factor in the development of COPD (85-90% of COPD deaths are caused by smoking).[1] COPD and other conditions such as asthma, is a result of damaged or inflamed airways, restricting air intake. Emphysema and chronic bronchitis tend to co-exist, further impacting quality of life. The end result of which can be living with oxygen bottles and mechanical respiratory assistance.[1] A growing number of studies (reviewed below) support benefits of Tai Chi for alleviating symptoms of chronic respiratory disease, and may help compensate for damaged airways.

Tai Chi and forms of Qi Gong may also benefit upper respiratory conditions as well. In my own practice, if my sinuses are congested, by the end of Tai Chi or the Eight Treasures Breathing exercise, my sinuses open up completely and any congestion disappears. This may be due to enhanced blood flow through the sinus passages, which can reduce swollen sinuses. Auxiliary Qi Gong exercises which involve pounding the chest can also bring up congestive matter from the lungs, which allows the body to expel it easier.

Tai Chi More Than Doubled My Lung Function

"I was diagnosed with emphysema in 1994. Like many people, I was a shallow breather. Tai Chi breathing taught me how to exercise unused portions of my lungs and strengthen them. In 2000, a lung function test showed an increase from 17% to 47%."

- Walter (From *Energy Arts.com*).

Essentially, Tai Chi and many forms of Qi Gong, by maximizing optimal use of oxygen in the body, is a good thing for any condition, but particularly for chronic breathing diseases and conditions. An added benefit for smokers, aside from permitting more efficient oxygen exchange, may be effects on smoking cessation efforts as a result of enhanced states of mindfulness. Mindfulness of smoking cues and triggers can short circuit unconscious habitual behaviors and lead to smoking cessation (discussed more in the conclusion). Smoking cessation is the single most effective means to reduce the risk of COPD, or to slow the development of COPD.[1]

Meditative practices have long been used to create greater levels of awareness towards the cessation of addiction. Although meditation and mindfulness is often geared towards a more general behavioral perspective, such as addiction to negative thoughts, behaviors and relationships, such practices can also be valuable for all forms of self-destructive behaviors. Tai Chi was used with great success in a smoking cessation program at the University of Miami.[3] Participants experienced an overall smoking cessation rate of 83%.

I have had three of my own students tell me they quit smoking due to Tai Chi, as a result of becoming more aware and in control of their smoking habits. One student even stated that until they took the Tai Chi class, they had never before contemplated quitting smoking. Tai Chi as a mindfulness based practice is described further in the conclusion, which explains how Tai Chi and other forms of moving meditation can be used to gain greater control and awareness of addictions and addictive behavior.

Studies on Tai Chi, Asthma, and COPD

Dr. Chenchen Wang, with the Division of Rheumatology at Tufts Medical Center, conducted an extensive review on the effects of Tai Chi for patients with various chronic conditions.[4] Benefits were reported for cardiovascular and respiratory functions, in addition to benefits for flexibility, immunity, strength, arthritis symptoms, and psychological effects. The main drawback identified was a lack of theoretical foundations regarding the mechanism of benefit.

Tai Chi Regulated My Lung Function

"I suffer with a chronic lung condition called cystic fibrosis. This affects the mucus membrane of the lungs and clogs the airways of the lungs, shrinking lung capacity and making breathing short or difficult. It also affects the processes of the digestive system which is not able to absorb nutrients properly. Often intravenous antibiotics are required to help maintain good lung function. When I had done my first Tai Chi class I felt so refreshed, vitalized and happy that I decided to come along and join in on a regular basis. The following week I returned to the class and have continued to do so since right up to the present day. The benefits of attending a Tai Chi class are many. My lung function has increased by 200ml and my weight has increased. My overall health is fantastic, considering I have cystic fibrosis. I use Tai Chi daily to help with coping with cystic fibrosis, regulating my lung function. All in all Tai Chi has saved my life."

- Karl (From *Mindful Tai Chi. Testimonials*).

The theory of Metarobics may present the missing link, as a mechanism related to a state of dynamic physiological relaxation combined with slow deep breathing, as exercises which enhance blood oxygen saturation and diffusion, through an unrestricted vasculature. Enhanced physiological functioning benefits all mechanisms of the body, including a beneficial increase in associated t-lymphocytes and the various chemicals and hormones within the body (see Chapter 6 for more on the role of Tai Chi in immunity).

Other studies have supported the benefits of Tai Chi for COPD, through improved lung function and tolerance for activity. One particularly large study involved 206 COPD patients, which were randomly assigned to one of three groups – a Tai Chi group, a walking group (combined with a focus on breathing), and a non-exercise control group.[5] The Tai Chi group experienced significant improvements on the six minute walk test and in breathing capacity, as well as for COPD condition. The walking group had no change in condition or measurements, while the non-exercise control group experienced a decline in function on all measures.

A smaller scale study investigated the effects of Tai Chi on pulmonary function (lung volume and lung capacity) in asthmatic children.[6] Fifteen children were enrolled into a twelve week Tai Chi program, and compared to 15 who did not do Tai Chi. All children in both groups had comparable levels of pulmonary function and severity of asthmatic symptoms before the start of the program. At the conclusion of the program, the children in the Tai Chi group experienced significant improvement in pulmonary function, compared to no change in the children who did not do Tai Chi. The Tai Chi group also reported benefits for asthmatic symptoms.

Tai Chi practice has been documented to result in significant improvements in peak flow (amount of air which can be pushed from the lungs), as well as asthma control and quality of life measurements.[7] Asthma patients were also able to increase maximum oxygen consumption. Tai Chi was noted as a potential effective non-drug adjunct therapy for those with persistent asthma, based on research findings. A growing body of research supports a variety of benefits for people with breathing disorders.

From a more purely Metarobic perspective, related to reversing hypoxia, it should be noted that even as early as 1967, researchers observed that hypoxia may play a role in asthma symptoms, as a result of narrowing airways.[8] Acute attacks can result in uneven ratios in the amount of air reaching the alveoli in the lungs, compared to the perfusion of blood reaching the alveoli (small balloon like structures where oxygen exchange takes place). The researchers believe that this may result in arterial hypoxia more often than had been previously noted. It is interesting to note that oxygen is administered to asthmatics to alleviate hypoxia, if blood oxygen saturation falls below 92%.

It would be worth studying any effects Metarobic exercises may have on the ventilation-perfusion ratios of oxygen in the alveoli, and reversal of hypoxia. A recent overview of Hypoxemia (abnormally low concentration of oxygen in the blood) in patients with COPD notes that as symptom severity increases, so does hypoxia and hypoxemia.[9] Long term oxygen therapy has been shown to improve conditions in patients with severe hypoxemic respiratory failure, but the authors state that optimal treatment for patients is uncertain. It might be hoped that Tai Chi Therapy may prove to be one such optimal treatment, pending further research.

Yangsheng Qi Gong[10] has been used in China as a form of therapy for bronchial asthma. A six month study of 30 asthma patients found significant benefits from these exercise on the amount of air which can be expelled from the lungs. Lower levels of peak airflow is an indication of constricted airways. Benefits were also found for reduced rates of hospitalization, fewer sick days from work, reduced antibiotic use, as well as lower rates of emergency treatment, compared to a control group which received standard care.

Since inflammation is also prevalent with these diseases, Metarobic exercises, as a potential anti-inflammatory, may also help provide relief inflammation associated with asthma and other chronic lower respiratory diseases (see Chapter 6: *Metarobics for Immunity, Diabetes, and Pain* for more details on the anti-inflammatory effects of Tai Chi).

Tai Chi Helps My Asthma Attacks

"As an asthma sufferer for many years, I find Tai Chi helpful in many ways. While concentrating on relaxed abdominal breathing with open and closing hands, slowing my breathing down, and using imagery to relax my mind, along with relaxing shoulders, I find I can reduce an attack in most situations."

– Chris (from *Tai Chi for Health Institute*)

Chapter 6

Metarobics for Immunity, Diabetes and Pain

Enhancing Qualify of Life

As noted earlier, the Metarobic response resulting from exercises such as Tai Chi and various forms of Qi Gong has been shown to have a direct effect on the immune system, beyond what is experiences with conventional exercise. Influenza (the flu) is the eighth leading cause of death in the United States (primarily resulting in deaths among older adults due to a compromised immune system). According to the Center for Disease Control (CDC), 90 percent of deaths from influenza occur in those 65 years of age or older.[1]

As people age the thymus (located in front of the heart) shrinks, and can become non-functional in your sixties or seventies. The thymus is a gland which, aside from producing various hormones, also plays a vital role in the development of T-lymphocytes (or T-cells). T-cells are a type of white blood cell which protects the body from bacteria and viruses.

Tai Chi – Sick Less And Sleep Better

Paul, a student at Fullerton College, was very dedicated to the practice of Tai Chi. Realizing the benefits of Tai Chi and the Eight Treasures, he religiously performed these exercises daily. Ten years later, he stated that since practicing Tai Chi, he has never been sick, even when in continuous contact with those who had whatever cold or flu was going around. He did mention that on days he had been overly busy, and missed a few days when around friends or family who were sick, he would feel the beginnings of a cold coming on. This would prompt Paul back to daily practice – and the cold would disappear. This happened often enough that he realized that there did indeed seem to be something behind the rumored benefits of Tai Chi and Qi Gong for enhanced immunity. Paul finally came to the point that even when he retired at a late hour (even 2:00 or 3:00 at night), he would do at least some Tai Chi or Qi Gong. Even when exhausted, he could feel energy returning. He also found that Tai Chi helped him fall asleep faster. Paul stated that it was almost as if his mind began entering a sleep like state during his Tai Chi practice.

Hypoxia has been identified as one possible cause for age related decline in the immune system.[2] Researchers believe that the immune system can be manipulated with drugs to influence oxygen and assist those with poor immune systems, or possibly in some circumstances help with autoimmune diseases and conditions. Since Tai Chi enhances blood oxygen saturation and diffusion, Metarobic exercises may have a similar effect without having to resort to medications, which can have dangerous side effects (keeping in mind to never change your medications without consulting with your doctor).

Studies on the effects of Tai Chi practice on immunity provides support for this. Researchers at the University of Illinois noted that high intensity exercises (such as high impact aerobics) can result in short term immune suppression, despite long term benefits for cardiovascular health.[3] The study showed that in comparison, Tai Chi practice enhanced immunity with short and long term beneficial effects.

Dr. Jennifer Robbins, with the Department of Internal Medicine at the University of Cincinnati, cites numerous studies which demonstrate that hypoxia has a negative effect on proliferation and release of T cells.[4] T Cells are important for mucosal defense, immunity, and for fighting inflammation. Dr. Robbins notes that hypoxic areas have been measured in lymph nodes, areas of inflammation, wounds, solid tumors, and bone fractures, as well as in joints with rheumatoid arthritis. The author and her colleagues state that hypoxia inhibits channels in T cells which are required for normal lymphocyte activation.

Tai Chi For A Disease Free, Pain Free Life

"I am convinced that Tai Chi has helped me with the Hepatitis C virus in my body, and has helped with my immune system to prevent damage. I had been losing hope until I started Tai Chi. I have also been migraine free and headaches are a thing of the past. It is wonderful to be free of that chronic pain, and my energy levels and outlook on life are up. I feel that Tai Chi and my more holistic lifestyle is helping my immune system. I am able to do more after a year of Tai Chi, and I end class with a wonderful sense of well-being (I used to fall into a deep sleep, exhausted). By making Tai Chi a priority, I hope to decrease the Hepatitis C symptoms as much as possible. Years after starting Tai Chi, and doing it daily, I have benefited in ways I could not imagine. Medical tests have improved, liver pain is gone, as are muscle and joint discomfort. It has given me my life back!"

– Wendy (From *Wendy's Wellness Website*).

Tai Chi practice has been shown to have beneficial effect on T cells.[5] In a study on the effects of 12 weeks of Tai Chi practice, regulatory T Cells had significantly increased. Monocytes (large white blood cells) also decreased significantly. Lower Monocyte counts are an indication of good health, since Monocytes increase in response to infection and chronic inflammation, indicating poor health.

Overall, the research on Tai Chi supports specific benefits for improved mucosal defense and a lower risk of autoimmune and inflammatory disorders.[5] The reasons for this were undetermined, although the researchers suggested that benefits may be due to the overall health benefits of exercise. The theory of Metarobics suggests that beyond the general benefit of exercise, Metarobic based exercises such as Tai Chi may have specific effects related to enhanced blood oxygen saturation, diffusion, effects on oxygen based metabolism, and reversal of hypoxia.

It is worth noting that vigorous exercise for 90 minutes or more can result in adverse changes to the immune system, while there have been mixed reports as to the benefits of moderate aerobic exercise on antibody production.[5] This may be a result of the oxygen supply of the body being commanded by the large muscle groups during aerobic exercise, and a resulting oxygen deficit during prolonged exercise in the other organs of the body (again, as indicated by stomach cramps when exercising after eating).

Research has also looked at the effects of Tai Chi practice on virus specific lymphocytes. A study examining the effects of Tai Chi on varicella zoster (Shingles) virus specific lymphocytes, found a significant increase in these lymphocytes as a result of 15 weeks of Tai Chi training in a group of older adults.[6] The Tai Chi group experienced an almost 50% increase in cell mediated immunity to varicella zoster virus, despite not receiving the vaccine, compared to no change in a comparison group. A third group received the shingles vaccine, which resulted in a 75% increase.

Another study found that when the vaccine was given to a Tai Chi group, they experienced a 173% increase in antibodies at the three week measure, compared to a 58% increase in a control group which did not do Tai Chi, but also received the vaccine.[3] At the 6 week post-vaccine measure, the Tai Chi group had a 130% increase in antibodies (compared to 54% in the non Tai Chi group), and a 109% increase at the 20 week follow up (compared to 10% in the non Tai Chi group). This indicates the importance of vaccination, but also demonstrates the benefit of Tai Chi for enhancing overall immunity. The researchers noted that Tai Chi may be particularly valuable for those diseases for which there is no vaccine.

It Took Two Heart Attacks And A Tai Chi Class To Be Disease Free

"In 2002 I had a heart attack. This followed with four years of flu, bronchitis, and pneumonia. Then I had a second heart attack. I then started Tai Chi, and for the last two years I have not had a cold, flu, pneumonia, or bronchitis, and less occurrence of angina. I am convinced that my health will continue to improve as I practice Tai Chi."

– Bruce. (From *Tai Chi for Health Institute Newsletter*).

The risk and severity of shingles increases with age, as the result of a decline in immunity to the varicella zoster virus. The amount of decline in immunity varies considerably from one older adult to the next, which may be due to differences in physical and emotional functioning. Psychological stress in older adults can result in the occurrence of herpes zoster, and depression can result in a reduction in immunity to shingles.[6] Aside from direct physiological benefits on immunity, Tai Chi can also have direct effects on stress and depression (discussed briefly in the conclusion), through the mindfulness based component as a form of moving mediation.

One last area to consider related to the practice of Qi Gong (breathing exercises) and Metarobic effects relates to an exercise called the "Marrow Washing Exercise." Bone marrow is responsible for stem cells, which can develop into the red blood cells, which carry life giving oxygen throughout the body. Scientists are coming to realize that the bone marrow may play a large role in the bodies healing abilities.[7] Scientists at King's College in London have been investigating the powerful effect on healing of a protein called HMGB1, which is secreted in the body by immune cells.[7] This protein was used as a catalyst to activate stem cells in the bone marrow.

Dr. John McGrath, one of the researchers, noted HMGB1 acts as a catalyst, awakening stem cells lying dormant in the body's bone marrow, and may have a dramatic impact on everything from treating people with rare genetic illnesses to burns and ulcers. Tai Chi and other Metarobic exercises may activate HMGB1 and other healing proteins, supporting the "marrow washing" reputation of these exercises.

Tai Chi For Mental And Physical Health

"I have had unstable emotions for more than 30 years. Now, since Tai Chi class, I am about 80% better. I am able to feel emotions without feeling as overwhelmed. In the past, I have also had symptoms of chronic fatigue syndrome. This has gone on for many years, and I felt ill more often than I felt well. Now I have much better energy and stamina, and I am sick much less often."

— Steve (From *Orange County Tai Chi Studio. What Our Tai Chi Students Say*)

The theory of Metarobics adds to a better understanding of how and why Tai Chi benefits immunity. Current understanding of benefits in research on Tai Chi is primarily limited to relaxation and stress reduction, and effects of stress on the body (as well as benefits as a mild form of aerobic exercise).[6] Understanding the effects of enhanced blood oxygen saturation and diffusion, impact on hypoxia (oxygen deficiency) and enhanced metabolic function takes this understanding one step further.

A compromised immune system can leave one vulnerable to autoimmune diseases, illness and infection, as well as put one at an increased risk for cancer. Based on the wide diversity of conditions which exercises such as Tai Chi and forms of Qi Gong have been documented to benefit, it may be possible that these exercises boost every system of the body, including the immune system.

Metarobics and Diabetes

Diabetes is a complex condition affected by many variables, consisting of a group of metabolic diseases which affect blood sugar. It can occur as a result of the pancreas not producing enough insulin, or as a result of cells not responding to the insulin that is produced. The main forms of diabetes are type one diabetes, in which the body cannot produce insulin, and type two diabetes, in which the body becomes resistant to insulin. Type 2 diabetes is almost always preceded by "pre-diabetes," in which blood glucose levels are higher than normal, but not high enough to be diagnosed as diabetes (but can still be damaging to the heart and circulatory system, and puts one at risk for type 2 diabetes).[8]

Diabetes is considered a metabolic disorder, resulting from the way the body uses digested food for energy.[9] As a metabolic disorder, it can be hoped that exercises such as Tai Chi may indeed have a true metabolic effect via the Metarobic action described in chapters one and two (with hope of either helping or preventing diabetes). However, there are many complications to the disease, as well as underlying factors which will necessitate a larger body of research to truly understand effects of these exercises on diabetic conditions.

Tai Chi Helped Control My Diabetes And Glaucoma

"I felt depressed, unhappy and stressed. I could not seem to get good control of my Type 2 diabetes. Then a friend introduced me to Tai Chi, and it was a perfect fit. I loved to move, and it made me feel peaceful. Then a pleasant surprise came. My A1C test for glucose control came back as high normal, less than 6%, compared to my past results which were over the target level of 7%. I also had been having a problem with glaucoma, but it is now under control and my vision has improved. I feel it is all because of Tai Chi."

– Sharon (From *Dr Lam's Tai Chi, Health & Lifestyle Newsletter. What Tai Chi Means to Me*).

The theory of Metarobics indicates potential avenues of investigation, which may at least show promise for helping with the condition. It should be kept in mind that type 1 and type 2 diabetes can occur for a variety of reasons, including genetic defects, pancreatic diseases, certain drugs or chemicals, infections, and other conditions. As such, Tai Chi and other Metarobic type exercises may have limited direct effects on at least some forms of diabetes.

Some scientists are researching possible links between certain viruses and diabetes,[8,10] in which case if Tai Chi can help the body combat viruses as a whole, then there may be some preventive effect via a secondary approach. Also, type 2 diabetes has been primarily linked to physical inactivity, obesity and being overweight. Exercise (including exercise such as walking or Tai Chi) and losing body weight are identified by the American Diabetes Association as two of the best ways of lowering risk for type 2 diabetes.[9] As a mindfulness based exercise, Tai Chi may have the added benefit for weight loss by enhancing conscious awareness of eating habits and triggers.

Potential benefits of Tai Chi related to hypoxia (oxygen deficiency) and diabetes may relate to the interactions between hyperglycemia (high blood sugar) and hypoxia, and may also affect diabetic retinopathy (damage to the retina which can lead to blindness). Hyperglycemia and hypoxia can affect cytosolic and mitochondrial free NADH (an enzyme involved with metabolic pathways and linked to diabetic complications).[11] Combined, these two risk factors for blindness accelerate diabetic retinopathy and other complications of diabetes, by augmenting metabolic pathways fueled by free NADH.

Vascular disease can affect retinal blood flow and associated delivery of glucose and oxygen. Poor glycemic control can result in worsening of diabetic eye disease as a result of an interaction between hyperglycemia and hypoxia.[11] The main points of interest is that hypoxia, or oxygen deficiency, is once more a culprit in poor health outcomes. This indicates the importance of investigating potential effects of Metarobic type exercises such as Tai Chi on hypoxic conditions.

I Lost Weight And My Pre Diabetic Condition

"I was diagnosed as pre diabetic, and was told by my doctor that I needed to lose a lot of weight. I was so obese I could not walk unaided. I started Tai Chi, and over time was able to walk without aids, and began losing weight. I was retested and was no longer pre diabetic. I have been doing Tai Chi for over four years now, and have lost so much weight and increased my fitness that I am now swimming and working out at the gym as well."

– Cheryl (From *Tai Chi for Health Institute. What Inspired Me to Start Tai Chi*).

Further support, suggesting a need for investigating Metarobic exercises for enhanced oxygen use in the body, relates to metabolic changes resulting from diabetes. These metabolic changes can decrease cardiac efficiency and result in reduced tolerance to oxygen-limited conditions.[12] Metarobic exercises may or may not prevent these metabolic changes as a result of diabetes, but it would be worth investigating if Metarobic exercises enhance cardiac efficiency and tolerance to oxygen-limited conditions, and any differences from conventional exercise.

Another factor to consider is the death of insulin producing pancreatic cells, which is tied directly to the development of diabetes. Can Tai Chi and similar Metarobic exercises prevent or halt pancreatic cell death? There is no research on the effects of Tai Chi or related exercises on pancreatic cell death to date, but research has been conducted showing that reduced oxygenation (hypoxia) is an important cause of cell loss and transplant failure in pancreas transplants in diabetic patients.[13]

Aside from further suggesting that oxygen deficiency may play a role in a wide range of illnesses and physiological malfunction, including diabetes, these findings also indicate that Metarobic exercises may help reduce risk of transplant organ rejection. Organs are particularly sensitive to hypoxia. Metabolic support is provided for donor organs, in order to enhance oxygen carrying capacity.[13] By enhancing blood oxygen diffusion and saturation, Metarobic exercises may help combat the risk of hypoxia following organ transplant.

Metarobics for Pain and Inflammation

One of the constants that has run throughout the personal stories on the benefits of Tai Chi that I have come across, is the impact of Tai Chi and forms of Qi Gong on pain. From a Metarobic perspective this seems logical, since it makes sense that a more efficiently operating body can deal better with pain and illness, and would be able to more effectively generate natural pain relievers such as cannabinoids (so called due to its effects on the body, which are similar to marijuana or cannabis).

Four Classes and the Pain was Gone

"Since being diagnosed with rheumatoid arthritis I struggled with performing any type of physical activity. Even something as simple as a leisurely stroll would leave me in a great amount of pain. Then I read that the Arthritis Foundation recommended Tai Chi as a "natural answer to exercise for those with arthritis." I tried a Tai Chi class and after an hour I was hooked. After only four classes I began to notice an improvement in my joints. On a whim I decided to go for a walk one day, and to my surprise, I ended up walking four miles. Even more surprising was that I experienced no joint pain the following day."

– Heather (From *Rosewell Tai Chi. Testimonials*).

Cannabinoids are a natural chemical the body secretes which accounts for the "runners high," along with endorphins, which is the body's version of morphine. Cannabinoids are a compound produced in the body which helps regulate the systems in the body, ranging from the immune and nervous system to the digestive system.[14] Since there is evidence that Tai Chi boosts the various healing agents in the body, as evidenced by the studies mentioned throughout this book, it is no surprise that these exercises would have similar effects on the generation of natural pain relieving chemicals in the body. Benefits which do not carry the risk of death and addiction which their illegal counterparts carry.

Research conducted at the Proteomic Core Laboratory is among the first to examine effects of Tai Chi on a molecular level, including effects on proteins affecting inflammation.[15] Proteins are large molecules consisting of one or more chains of amino acids, which perform many functions within the body, including catalyzing metabolic functions. It is estimated that there are as many as 50,000 different types of proteins in the human body.

In this study, the effect of Tai Chi practice on 18 proteins following Tai Chi were examined. Significant differences were found following Tai Chi practice, including a decrease in compliment factor B, indicating low levels of inflammation in the body (levels of complement factor B are high when there is inflammation in the body). An increase in compliment factor H was also found, which are proteins associated with the prevention of vascular damage and degeneration of the macula (the macula is the part of the eye responsible for detailed central vision).[15]

Hypoxia is also implicated in pain and inflammation. Low blood oxygen saturation levels can increase feelings of pain. Nurses can confirm a patient's pain intensity by measuring blood oxygen saturation with an oximeter. Lower levels of oxygen tend to correspond with increased pain. One form of pain caused by too little blood flow is called claudication.[16] Claudication generally affects the legs, but can also affect the arms as well.

This condition is generally a result of peripheral artery disease, due to clogging of the arteries and reduced blood flow in the arms or legs. Tai Chi and other Metarobic exercises may help claudication by gently increasing blood flow in the affected areas. Again, it would be important to document not only unique physiological mechanisms of action, but also differences, if any, from other exercise in these benefits

---

Before Tai Chi I Couldn't Walk

"Before taking the Tai Chi class, I couldn't walk a half mile, it hurt so much just to put my hands over my head. Sleeping was difficult, and there was no joy to life. I was an entire mess from head to foot. Medication, physical therapy, and swimming did not help. Then I heard about the Tai Chi study. I didn't know Tai Chi from a sneeze, but I figured I would get to meet people and it would get me out of the house. I didn't believe any of it. I thought this is so minimal, it's stupid. But after a few weeks, I began to feel better, and after 12 weeks the pain had diminished 90%. I have kept with Tai Chi, have lost 50 pounds, and can now walk three to seven miles a day. I wouldn't say it's a cure. I will say it's an effective method for controlling pain."

- Mary (one of the participants in Dr. Wang's study below).

Another area of research related to hypoxia is the effect of high altitude low oxygen environments on pain.[17] Experiments conducted with an expedition group of mountaineers yielded some interesting results. Under normal conditions, the expedition group had high pain thresholds, but at higher altitudes their pain thresholds decreased. Hypoxia was noted as the main cause.[17]

Dr. Chenchen Wang, a researcher at Tufts Medical Center, conducted a study on the effects of Tai Chi on fibromyalgia, a chronic pain condition.[18] After 12 weeks participants in the Tai Chi group experienced significant improvements in pain, fatigue, physical functioning, sleeplessness and depression, compared to a group which performed stretching and received classes in wellness education. Pain relieving effects were so significant, that one third of the participants in the Tai Chi group stopped using any form of pain medication.

Tai Chi has also been found to have a positive effect on tension headaches.[19] Researchers concluded that the effects of Tai Chi on pain levels might be the result of Tai Chi reducing stress. But based on the theories and research in this book, it also seems possible that the physiological effects on pain are related to enhanced circulation, as well as enhanced blood oxygen saturation and diffusion, which may boost the body's natural pain killers (such as the cannabinoids and endorphins mentioned above), either through more effective diffusion or production.

This is supported by a comparison study in Korea, which found significantly less pain and less body stiffness after 12 weeks of Tai Chi practice, as well as an improvement in balance.[20] The control group, which did not do Tai Chi, experienced no improvement. Some participants in the non Tai Chi group actually deteriorated in physical functioning.

Tai Chi has also been found to have an effect on rheumatoid arthritis. Rheumatoid arthritis is a chronic inflammatory disease which affects the musculoskeletal system, and can have different effects on different people, including chronic pain. It can come and go, and in its most severe form can lead to serious joint damage and disability. It can even affect other parts of the body. Inflammation occurs as the result of white blood cells attacking the body's own joint tissue.[21] As such, rheumatoid arthritis is an auto-immune disease, where the immune system attacks the body.

No one knows why this happens, but many studies on the effects of Tai Chi have demonstrated significant improvement in various symptoms, including pain. One of these studies recruited fifteen patients from a rheumatology department to practice Tai Chi twice a week for 12 weeks. Participants experienced significant improvements in lower-limb muscle function, as well as less pain, number of swollen joints, improved balance, and more confidence in moving.[22]

Other conditions which can result in chronic pain include Multiple Sclerosis. Multiple sclerosis is a chronic disease which attacks the central nervous system (the brain, spinal cord, and optic nerves). Symptoms can range from numbness of the limbs to complete paralysis or loss of vision. Multiple sclerosis (or MS), is also thought to be an autoimmune disease, in this case attacking the nervous system. The exact cause is unknown, but it is suspected to be related to environmental factors and a genetic predisposition. MS results in damaged myelin, the fatty substance which surrounds and protects the nerve fibers, and can also damage the nerves themselves.[23]

MS Could Not Stand Up To My Tai Chi

"On my last visit to my doctor, she wanted to know what I was doing to have so much improvement in my MS. I told her I was doing Tai Chi. She said to keep up the good 'chi.'"

– Neva (From *Tai Chi for Everyone*)

The research into Tai Chi and multiple sclerosis has been limited primarily to benefits for balance, improvement in walking speed, flexibility, vitality and social and psychological factors,[24] but if Tai Chi and other Metarobic exercises enhance the body's systems, there may be benefits for pain and other symptoms of multiple sclerosis as well, as indicated above by Neva's story above.

One small scale pilot study enrolled eight secondary progressive multiple sclerosis patients into a Tai Chi/Qi Gong class, which also included self massage. Benefits increased with the amount of time Tai Chi was practiced at home.[25] One participant who practiced little (about 50 minutes per week), experienced almost no benefits. Those who practiced for approximately 200 to 400 minutes per week reported benefits including improvement in balance, reduction in feelings of "pins and needles," pain, fatigue, depression, stiffness of joints, as well as reduced numbness in fingers and feet. Improvements were also noted in some participants for increase in walking distance, balance, general well-being, concentration, ability to move legs, and fine motor control.

Yoga Helped With Muscle Control for MS

I have multiple sclerosis, an auto immune disorder. Around 20 years ago I began losing the use of my muscles. Many rounds of doctors and hospitals later, and with no hope left, I tried a Yoga class. I am now starting to get some control over my muscles. Currently I cannot walk without help. My teacher is confident that I will be able to walk on my own in three years.

— Priya (From *The Health Site*)

The researchers noted that typical expectations of medical interventions is to slow the progression of the disease, which contrasted to reported benefits from doing Tai Chi, which actually showed improvements in functioning on several points. An over 31 % improvement in symptoms was reported. Replication of the study on a larger scale was recommended to better understand potential benefits, particularly considering the wide variety of symptoms associated with Multiple Sclerosis.[25]

Chapter 7

Essential Elements of Metarobics and Tai Chi for Therapy

Teaching, Learning and Researching Tai Chi and Qi Gong for Health

Tai Chi is fast becoming a popular exercise, resulting in a wide range of teaching methods. Some changes are beneficial, but others may reduce or even eliminate the unique benefits of Tai Chi. This chapter will provide a brief overview of the development of Tai Chi for health, and discuss what to look for in a Tai Chi class to maximize the benefits of Tai Chi from a Metarobic and structural perspective. This chapter will close with recommendations for effective research on Tai Chi and related exercises.

Tai Chi for Health

"Dr. Paul Lam is one of the pioneers who has worked hard to make Tai Chi user friendly for health. Dr. Lam started Tai Chi over 30 years ago after graduating from medical school. As a teen he suffered from osteoarthritis, and by the time he graduated medical school his condition was so debilitating that he could not even carry a briefcase. Since then Tai Chi has changed his life. His arthritis became well controlled, and he attributes his good health and positive attitude to his dedicated Tai Chi practice."

– Dr. Paul Lam (From *Tai Chi for Health Institute*)

As with most of the research presented in this book, Tai Chi is the main focus, since it is more common and more familiar to people in the United States than Qi Gong. But both forms of these exercises share many commonalities, including slow relaxed movements, gentle stretching of the limbs, focus on deep breathing and good postural alignment. Since some forms of Qi Gong, particularly those developed for martial purposes do not necessarily follow this format, elements of other forms of Qi Gong which can be detrimental for health will also be touched on.

There are many colorful histories and legends regarding the origins of Tai Chi,[1,2] but the essence behind the slow spiraling movements lies in its origin as a martial art. The slow movements permitted a level of mastery over muscle tension and body structure that allowed more efficient use of muscular power, as well as increased sensitivity in controlling the movements of a "stiffer" opponent. The person who was more relaxed could feel the tension in the other person, allowing anticipation of movements and an ability to redirect attacks. Once a Tai Chi master made contact with a person, they had total control over an opponent. Tai Chi Chuan literally translates as "Grand Ultimate Fist," due to its effectiveness in combat when practiced as a martial art.

Over time people came to realize that Tai Chi was a valuable health exercise as well, since deep breathing and removing tension from the body has many valuable health benefits. Since this is also the goal of many Qi Gong exercises, Tai Chi has become classified as a form of Qi Gong, and has since been popularized primarily as a health exercise.

The Breath and Pace in Tai Chi

The breath is at the core of many of the health benefits of Tai Chi. Many people tend to breathe shallowly, expanding the ribs in what is called chest breathing, as opposed to diaphragmatic breathing, which involves expanding the stomach (activating the rib muscles and diaphragm). Most books on running or aerobic exercise are quick to point out the benefits of diaphragmatic breathing for increasing oxygen intake.[1] Diaphragmatic breathing is a hallmark of Tai Chi, which focuses on expanding the chest and abdomen to maximize inhalation of air. Indeed, some Tai Chi instructors also say to expand the back as well, which can result in expansion of the posterior ribs. During these exercises, breathing is done through the nose, rather than the mouth (assuming your nasal passages are clear). Nose breathing is considered healthier since it pre-warms and moistens the air as it comes through the nasal passages, and helps the body to trap and eliminate contaminants from the air before it reaches the lungs. Breathing through the mouth can result in more frequent respiratory infections. The Chinese have an interesting saying on this: "You would not try to stuff food up your nose, so why would you breathe through your mouth?"

Shallow breathing moves only a small fraction of the lungs total air volume into and out of the body (approximately 0.5 liters) with each breath. Deep breathing can increase lung capacity, and can increase air volume to three to five liters, depending on the lung capacity of the individual.[3] Being in its infancy, the field of Metarobics is ripe for research to determine exact effects. But in the meantime, the observations presented in this book provide a good start. If you find yourself completing several movements with one breath, slow down each movement to match the breath.

The goal is to completely fill the lungs during the first half of each movement, and completely empty the lungs by the end of each movement, as slowly as possible without feeling short of breath. You do not need to try to consciously match the breath to the movement – with time the breath will correspond naturally, without trying to force it. There is also some variation between movements.

Moving slowly, while focusing on being relaxed and breathing fully from the abdomen and chest, without overdoing it, will result in a natural rhythm without strain. If you feel you are running out of breath when going slow, speed up the movements. Alternatively, some practitioners suggest taking more than one breath during each movement (breathing in and out during the first half of a movement, and then again during its completion). For health, the important part is being slow and relaxed, with full comfortable breaths. Overall, I tell my students not to worry about the breath, since it tends to follow naturally with the movements. Over time your body will fall into a natural rhythm.

For martial practice, slower and faster paces may be used to train the body for specific goals for self-defense. For health, fast paces can enhance aerobic conditioning, but a slower pace enhances greater relaxation of muscle tension. A slower pace also works on a different perspective of balance. For health purposes, the guidelines for a slower pace have demonstrated the greatest increase in blood oxygen saturation and Metarobic effects.

Being "Single Weighted"

Another key element to maximize diffusion of the blood and oxygen throughout the body, as well as to develop a greater level of relaxation in the mind and body, may relate to the way the weight is carried by the legs. During almost every movement in Tai Chi, the goal is to be "single weighted," that is, the weight of the body is essentially balanced entirely over one leg or the other, shifting back and forth, as a person transitions through the movements.

When the weight of the body is balanced equally between the legs, a person is considered to be "double weighted." The reason for being single weighted lies in the martial origins of Tai Chi, but the practical effect for health is that by letting the weight of the body shift entirely to one leg (for example the right leg), the rest of the body can be allowed to relax entirely. Including the left leg (called the "empty leg"), the hips, the torso, shoulders, arms, neck and head. As the movement transitions through to the opposite leg (for example, to the left leg), the other side relaxes. An analogy is often made to the idea of imagining one leg being "full" of water, and the water "pouring" into the "empty" leg, as one shifts through to the next movement, until the full leg becomes empty, and the empty leg becomes full.

This transition between empty and full occurs throughout the entire form. Essentially Tai Chi is the act of balancing on one leg and then the other, while relaxing the opposite leg and the entire body. This is the reason why Tai Chi is such a valuable exercise for enhancing balance, and also works to strengthen the knees (providing the knees are kept aligned with the feet and are not over extended, to prevent knee strain).[4]

Balance And Knees, The Best of Both

"After two brain surgeries, I had constant severe headaches and suffered from loss of coordination and severe dizziness to the point of passing out. I friend told me that Tai Chi had improved her balance, so I decided to try it. Within two weeks the dizziness disappeared so much that I did not need to use the transderm scop patch I was dependent on. The headaches become less frequent and my coordination got better. Now I rarely experience any headaches. I also had torn the medial meniscus cartilage in both knees. I had the left knee operated on. I could not walk without knee braces, and could only walk slowly. Now I only wear the braces when I do Tai Chi. I can walk much faster and can get up and down the stairs to the subway with no problem or loss of balance."

– Victoria (From *Tai Chi Chuan Center. Testimonials*)

Weighting one leg, with the leg bent, also increases the heart rate slightly (although not to what is considered moderate aerobic levels). Research will need to determine if the weighted leg "robs" the body of blood oxygen saturation, since levels are lower during Tai Chi compared to standing Qi Gong poses with the legs straight. On the other hand, the weighted leg may enhance blood flow and diffusion throughout the body through osmotic pressure, more so than if the form were practiced in a standing position. During measurements of Tai Chi, and those

Qi Gong exercises which are performed with a bent kneed stance, blood oxygen saturation increases one to two points. During the standing poses of Qi Gong, it tends to increase two to three points.

With the large body of literature on the benefits of Tai Chi, it may be possible that the slightly faster heart rate from the bent kneed stance of Tai Chi may have particular benefits (beyond strengthening the knees and legs). Further research needs to determine if pure Qi Gong exercises such as the Eight Treasures provide even greater benefits, being focused for health as opposed to adapted from a martial routine. Try both of you have the time, since both have been proven to have benefits, and make your own observations. If you have a specific medical condition your doctor may have recommendations for practice as well.

Extending the Spine, Strengthening the Knees

One other critical element is the positioning of the spine during Tai Chi. As the movements are performed, the tailbone is tucked forward and the crown of the head is extended, as if a string were being pulled from the top of the head and the tip of the tailbone. This releases muscle tension in the shoulders and lower back, straightens the spine, and maximizes spinal rotation and adjustment. It is important however, not to strain or overdo the straightening of the back, particularly in the beginning. Moving too quickly beyond your usual range of movement may lead to back strain from unfamiliar positions, or to movement beyond the range of motion for your body. Over time, if practiced daily, you will find your back becomes more limber and less prone to back pain, and easier to straighten.[5]

Tai Chi – Better Back, Stronger Legs

"I started Tai Chi three years ago upon recommendations of my doctor. I suffered constant muscular pain all over my back, and it was suggested that it would be good for strengthening my lower back. I found I really enjoyed the low impact nature of the exercise, and I also found the meditation and relaxation aspects extremely beneficial. I was surprised at how disciplined I was with practice, and within one year all of my back pain was completely gone, as well as stiffness in my joints. My posture improved, my legs grew stronger, and I learned to release tension throughout my body, particularly my shoulders."

– Joyce. (From *Tai Chi for Health Institute*).

Other structural elements include benefits for the knees, as well as increased leg strength. During the poses and movements of Tai Chi and some postures of Qi Gong, you are essentially in a semi crouched stance, similar to exercises prescribed by physical therapists. The bent kneed stance during Tai Chi and many Qi Gong poses helps to strengthen the muscles of the legs and knees (with proper knee and foot alignment, preventing the knee from extending past the foot). Before I started Tai Chi, I had chronic knee problems. My knees were swollen and crackly, and got to the point that I had to give up running. Over time, the stance training of Tai Chi developed the muscles around my knees, including a band of muscle at the back of the knee which wraps around and supports the knee joint. I no longer have knee pain and can now run pain free.

An article I read when I first started Tai Chi over 25 years ago, stated that Tai Chi practice can develop the knee muscles to the point that they will take about 85% of the weight off of the knee joint. Essentially, the developed muscles of the knee can act as a natural knee brace. This is one more area in need of further research, but theoretical elements and personal accounts indicate another promising benefit for health.

Miscellaneous Elements

When practicing Tai Chi, aside from slow relaxed movements, full breaths, slightly bent knees and a straight spine, a few other details should be kept in mind. To maximize relaxation in the arms and shoulders, let the shoulders drop and relax. The hands, except in specific instances such as "crane spreads its wings" (which can also vary according to style), never rise above the head, nor do they extend totally straight. In most movements the active arm is curved gently. Over-extending results in tension. The hands should be relaxed as well, with a slight counter tension to counteract years of gripping the hands in stress and tension, by pressing the palm down as if on a table.

On the other hand, some schools of Tai Chi let the non-active hand hang totally relaxed at the side. This is yet another area in need of research, to determine any differences in benefits resulting from a totally relaxed hand, compared to gently pressing down. Pressing down may counter years of tension and open up the circulation in the hands. However, letting the hand hang relaxed may help generate deeper states of relaxation.

An exercise I have my Tai Chi students do at the beginning of the semester is to have them stand with their hands relaxed at their sides. Most students' hands curl inward like claws, which is the result of years of tension, like the picture on page 31. As mentioned above, the tension in the hands can be stretched out and relaxed by pressing down as if on an invisible table during the form. This can also open up the capillaries in the hands, which is felt as a pleasant tingling or buzzing sensation in the hands.

The accuracy of the individual movements (such as "crane spreads its wings," or "part the horse's mane") may be less critical than the general form and method of each movement. If practicing Tai Chi as a martial art, it is important to hold the hands in an exact position, but for health and relaxation, observing key elements can generate most if not all of the benefits of Tai Chi practice, even if the hands or postures are not quite exact.

As outlined above, these key elements include relaxing the shoulders, arms and body, while tucking the hips and keeping the spine straight, gently bent knees aligned with the feet, and slow movements coupled with relaxed diaphragmatic breathing. Removing tension from the body while generating a focused yet relaxed and calm mental state are key goals of Tai Chi for health. Tai Chi as a martial art can take a lifetime to master, but the principles for health can be practiced immediately with an appropriate teacher or even DVD (see my website *Metarobics.com* for resources).

As a traditional Yang Style Tai Chi practitioner, it took me years to accept this conclusion. From a traditional format, it can take years or even decades before one can say they have mastered Tai Chi. But years of observation, research, and teaching support that the basic form of Tai Chi for health can be learned within a very short time. You can imagine how long it would have taken running or aerobics to become popular if you were told that before you could do the full exercise, you would have to spend one to two years learning individual movements.

What to Look for in a Tai Chi Class

To learn or practice Tai Chi for health, teaching ability can make more difference than the years of experience a teacher has in Tai Chi (something also hard to admit, as a long time practitioner). There are many traditionalists with a more martial orientation, who may have incredible skill in Tai Chi, but little patience as a teacher. One of the largest barriers to learning Tai Chi identified in a survey of major programs in the United States was lack of patience on the part of the instructor.[6]

An experienced teacher with a focus on Tai Chi for health often knows what to look for to enhance benefits for each person, and may be more proficient at adapting to student needs (while always keeping in mind the advice of your doctor). A third caveat is that some teachers, having learned in the old school master/disciple format, may be so invested in the way they were taught, that any adaptation is impossible. In the traditional format, it can take years before one can perform the full Tai Chi form.

Due to the variation in teaching styles, as well as styles of Tai Chi and Qi Gong, it is recommended to check out *all* of the classes in your area, to get an idea of what is available. Sometimes convenience is key. On the other hand, finding a group that you identify with may be more important. Find out what forms of Qi Gong and Tai Chi are practiced, and then do some research on the internet if no other resources are available. Talk with the students if you can, and find out what benefits they feel they are getting.

You may also wish to ask the teacher how long it takes to learn the form. A three month to two year learning curve is typical, but there may be auxiliary exercises or segments you can practice at home (this is why I developed the resources at *Metarobics.com*, to allow immediate practice of Tai Chi and the Eight Treasures Exercise). If you can try out a few classes, this might allow you to find out if the instructor has the qualities which will enhance your learning.

A Life Of Work Left Me In Pain. Until Tai Chi

"I used to work at a dry cleaner, ironing clothing all day long. Because of my job, I had developed arthritis in my hands. My fingers were swollen and in pain much of the time. After taking up Tai Chi, my fingers are no longer swollen or in pain, and I can move them without any problem. I now find myself doing house chores for a long period of time with ease, moving things around, picking them up, bending down and reaching up. I used to have to be careful about pushing myself because I would get muscle aches and headaches. But now I get a deeper than usual night's sleep, which feels really good. Also, recently my doctor said my bone density had increased by about 20% from three years ago. He was very surprised."

– Lun (From *Tai Chi Chuan Center. Testimonials*).

In a national survey of Tai Chi programs, being patient and adaptable were two of the most important attributes students identified for a Tai Chi teacher (even more so than knowledge of Tai Chi).[6] Use the principles outlined in this chapter as a guideline, and ask students in the class what benefits they have received from taking Tai Chi. If you are looking primarily for health, check to see whether the school stresses the health or martial aspects. Surprisingly, a large number of instructors still teach Tai Chi from a martial perspective (although this is valuable for those interested in the martial arts, as well as to preserve the complete art).

One school I observed had students (even the older ones, who were in their 70's) smash their shoulders against each other to practice a technique called "shoulder stroke." It is common in Chen style Tai Chi to raise the leg and then stomp the foot with great impact onto the ground. This may help develop skills for throwing an opponent, but is questionable regarding the health of the knee. Some schools practice a two person exercise called pushing hands, which can have some specific benefits for enhancing relaxation, but can also involve throws.

Gentle forms of push hands can be a good exercise to learn how to release tension in the body. A person may not realize how much muscle tension they actually have until they practice the push hands exercise with a more relaxed and experienced Tai Chi practitioner. Doing push hands exercises with a more experienced practitioner can help you to feel and better understand the tension in your body. But push hands exercises can also be taken to more extreme forms, which can include joint locks and throws. So watch a class or two, talk to the students, and check out as many classes as you can. Usually students are eager to share the benefits they have received, and this may be your best clue as to the effectiveness of the class for health.

Most Tai Chi and Qi Gong teachers are willing to accommodate the needs of their students, particularly if the student is respectful. As research and methods of teaching user friendly classes become more established, it will become easier to find classes and resources for Tai Chi and Qi Gong for health. One of the primary goals of this book is to help people rethink Tai Chi and associated exercises as a health exercise, one which can be as popular and accessible as any aerobics program.

For those who would like to enhance their teaching skills (being a master practitioner does not necessarily mean being a master teacher), teachers are encouraged to read Dr. Paul Lam's book *"Teaching Tai Chi Effectively,"* which is based on his more than 30 years of experience with Tai Chi, and experience teaching and training people to effectively lead classes for a variety of audiences.[7]

Although Qi Gong is usually taught in association with Tai Chi, a growing number of classes are focusing on forms of Qi Gong. When looking for Qi Gong classes, remember that Qi Gong can also include a wide range of practices. There are some unusual forms of folk Qi Gong which may be questionable regarding their health benefits (such as pressing the body against playground equipment to absorb youthful energy). Some forms of Qi Gong training involve holding poses for an hour or more, sometimes while visualizing movement of energy within the body.

The mind is a powerful thing, and there is some suggestion that visualizing energy patterns in the body may actually affect the brain and nervous system, sometimes in negative ways. Others have reported constipation or other intestinal disorders. On the other hand, many schools of Tai Chi and Qi Gong report using various visualizations to relax or direct healing in the body with beneficial effects. There are also forms of martial or hard Qi Gong, which can include practices with a focus on toughing the body – such as repeatedly striking the head with a heavy board. Practices can also involve striking the body with iron rods, or using reverse forms of breathing to toughen and pressurize the body, to make it impervious to blows (which can also raise blood pressure to dangerous levels). Although this might have enhanced some form of longevity in the days of hand to hand combat, in more modern times such exercises can be detrimental.

I know two Tai Chi practitioners who attributed severe health problems, including congestive heart failure, to the practice of reverse breathing during Tai Chi. Reverse breathing pressurizes the body to make it resistant to blows, but doing so through an entire Tai Chi or Qi Gong form may raise blood pressure to dangerous levels. Research will need to determine if even brief moments of reverse breathing has any benefit. From a theoretical perspective, holding the breath very briefly during some Qi Gong poses may momentarily increase blood pressure, with possible beneficial effects on strengthening blood vessel walls (based on the concept that brief moments of mild stress results in a positive response, similar to the effect of weight lifting on muscles).

Reverse breathing, conducted within certain parameters, may have similar effects, but it will take an extensive body of research to determine the relationship between time, damage, and any possible benefits. As a whole, I advocate following the natural mechanisms of the body, as well as discussing your practice with your doctor. Abdominal or diaphragmmatic breathing has been demonstrated as beneficial for health, as opposed to shallow upper chest breathing. It is the reason we have a diaphragm stretching across the bottom of our rib cage. This specialized muscle is specifically designed to maximize inhalation of the breath.

Until research can separate myth from fact and health from harm, the general recommendation is to focus on the basic health benefits of abdominal breathing, coupled with relaxation, and a gentle range of movement with good postural alignment (including the knees and feet). These basic principles underlie the most common practices and benefits of Tai Chi and Qi Gong for health. It can also be helpful to talk with the instructor, other students and your doctor, if you have questions or doubts regarding any practice.

Time will tell which Qi Gong practices are beneficial and which are rooted in folklore (although some folk practices do have many health benefits). The West has gone through a similar evolution. There are many questionable "health" practices in Western lore and traditions, such as rubbing goose droppings on the head to cure baldness. It is doubtful if such a practice would actually cure baldness, but the folk practice of using leaches to draw blood has made a comeback in the medical community.[8]

As time progresses, further research will help differentiate effective practices from folklore, but in the meantime, it is advisable for those interested in Tai Chi and Qi Gong to become as knowledgeable as possible. Learn the intent of any exercise you are considering, the evidence based rationale behind the benefits if known, and discuss your practice with a qualified doctor. There are many who feel strongly that many of the benefits of these exercises are unexplainable and beyond the known. But unique physiological responses indicate that many, if not all of the benefits of these exercises, are due to a physiological mechanism, one which can be measured and understood. This is the primary purpose of this book, to lay such a groundwork upon which to build.

Another at Deaths' Door

Before taking up Tai Chi, Master Jou Tsung Hwa developed a fondness for gambling. Combined with late hours at work, and playing hard afterwards, his abusive lifestyle resulted in an enlarged heart and prolapsed stomach by age 47. After visiting several doctors, he became despondent. Jou was told that there was no hope for repair to his heart, and surgery would be of only minor benefit for his stomach. Then a friend who was a long time Tai Chi practitioner convinced Jou to try Tai Chi. Within two weeks he began to feel better, and three years later tests showed that his stomach had healed. His heart has also returned to normal size, and all damage seemed to have disappeared. After seeing the cure that Tai Chi had enacted after conventional Western medicine failed, Jou Tsung Hwa became a teacher of Tai Chi. At age 81 he was still in good health, more active than many half his age, when he died an early death, when his car was hit by on oncoming van.

From *Taichifarm.org. The Grandmaster.*

This is not to discount the more esoteric practices and elements. As a long time practitioner, I have seen and experienced many unusual and unexplainable things. Even conventional exercises such as running have examples of the metaphysical and extraordinary (such as the "runner's high," which although many attribute to increased endorphins, also has advocates that something more is going on).[9] History is full of those who, having pushed their limits, have achieved something remarkable (which will be explored further in *Tai Chi – Mind, Body and Spirit*).

The primary benefits of most forms of Qi Gong, Tai Chi, and forms of Yoga which focus on relaxation and the breath, lies in the similarity of practices – slow relaxed, gentle movements, extending the range of motion without straining, coupled with deep breathing. The primary difference between Tai Chi and forms of Qi Gong and Yoga, is that Tai Chi is practiced moving (although some people, including myself, have developed stationary forms of Tai Chi, to make it more accessible for more people). Slow controlled movements which involve a shifting of weight, such as during Tai Chi practice, does have the added benefit for developing balance. Since death from falls is the leading cause of accidental death in older adults,[10] this can be a valuable aspect of Tai Chi practice.

Another barrier to learning Tai Chi for health is the long learning curve typical of most Tai Chi schools. Since Tai Chi originated as a martial art, it is often still taught from a long term master/disciple format, over a period of several years. The question I was finally forced to ask was, is it really necessary to have such a long learning curve to be able to use Tai Chi for health? When I began teaching Tai Chi at a community college, every semester I would have 20 to 30 new students. It was not unusual for students to take two semesters or more to learn the entire 24 style short form.

Tai Chi – The Breath of Life

"Five years ago I spent much of my days in bed or in a recliner. I was barely able to move without a walker. I developed asthma in my 40's, and also had rheumatoid arthritis, chronic migraines, chronic back and neck pain, as well as anxiety and depression. I had to retire and my doctor told me I would soon need a wheelchair. Then I remembered an article about Tai Chi. I signed up for a class, and after only three months I noticed a change in my mobility. I was able to transition from my walker to a cane, and was very excited. I was taking three 90 minute classes a week, and before long my pain and other symptoms improved. I even stopped having to take most of my asthma medications. Five years ago, I was on a walker and could not do anything. Now here I am teaching Tai Chi. It is phenomenal."

– Debbie (From *The Tampa Bay Times*).

Since many students were only taking the class one semester, and most would not continue practice beyond the class (at least until they got older and began to feel the effects of age), it seemed important that students should have a format which would introduce them to the entire form, to generate interest and enjoyment which might encourage later practice of Tai Chi as they got older.

It also seemed important to have something that could be practiced from the first week. So with a little trial and error, I found that it was possible to take a few minutes to introduce students to the ways of moving in Tai Chi, focusing first on the lower body, then the hands, and finally coordinating the two. Students were then able to follow through the entire form, by using various verbal cues. I used this format with great success over the next ten years, permitting instant practice of Tai Chi and the companion exercise Pa Duan Jin (the Eight Pieces of Silk Brocade, or the Eight Treasures Exercise). Looking at individual schools, I have found others who have successfully adapted teaching Tai Chi for immediate practice, but these were few and far between. Overall, Tai Chi seems to face an uphill battle before it becomes truly user friendly.

Tai Chi for Researchers

Researchers face a particular problem when it comes to researching Tai Chi. Methods, styles, and formats can differ so much from one instructor to the next, that it makes comparison difficult. One study may show significant benefits, and another may not, purely due to the style of Tai Chi or method of Tai Chi instruction. Compounding this difficulty is the format of most studies, which are completed anywhere in as short as five weeks to six months. Considering it can take one to two years to learn a Tai Chi form, what the researchers may end up measuring is learning Tai Chi as opposed to regular practice.

To overcome this shortcoming, researchers will either need to focus on those who already know Tai Chi, or use a format similar to the one I used in my college classes, so participants can begin practice of Tai Chi from the first class. Both formats bring difficulties. Tai Chi is not yet common enough for it to be easy to find a sufficient number of participants for most studies. There is also the question of style. Results from a fast paced Chen style form, as opposed to the slower Yang style, may generate very different results. Each form of Tai Chi may enhance health, but possibly from different perspectives.

It is critical to know the details of the form of Tai Chi being practiced – many contradictory results in research studies may be the result of different forms of Tai Chi being used, or different forms of instruction. One study noted that most of class time was spent in discussion.[11] As noted earlier, some forms of Tai Chi are more martial in format, with many fast and explosive movements, such as Chen style Tai Chi. The long learning curve typical of Tai Chi practice may also result in conflicting results from comparable studies (the latter being the reason I developed a Tai Chi Follow Along and Group Forms).

It needs to be determined if you will get the same benefits following Tai Chi as opposed to being able to practice it independently. Initial results from my own research indicates that physiological results may be similar if not the same, at least in regards to blood oxygen saturation and diffusion. The three students with cancer in my college classes used the follow along format, and felt that they had benefited tremendously. But to fully validate the benefits or differences between following Tai Chi, as opposed to independent practice, further research needs to be conducted. My experience indicates that results will be similar, but it is also likely that as one becomes more experienced with Tai Chi, a greater level of benefits will be derived, as indicated by the results of measurements in long time Tai Chi practitioners, presented in chapter one.

Until Tai Chi is popular enough that researchers can easily fill the numbers they need for their studies, or until a follow along format can be truly validated as being as effective as independent practice, researchers need to be very specific in the description of the format used. To truly replicate and validate studies on Tai Chi, several factors need to be detailed, including instructor experience, Tai Chi style, methods of instruction, focus of the class, and amount of time spent practicing in and out of class. It is not uncommon for more time to be spent in lecture and discussing elements of Tai Chi during class, as opposed to actual practice.[11]

But in the meantime, the growing abundance of research, even if lacking in details, still provides support for the many benefits of Tai Chi. The theories and understanding presented in this book will help shape a better understanding of Tai Chi and future avenues of research. To establish an understanding of the physiological effects of Tai Chi, particularly from a Metarobic perspective, it will be important to conduct studies which measure not just blood oxygen saturation and diffusion, but also effects on oxygen and blood perfusion within the internal organs, as well as possible effects on blood marrow production, protein synthesis, molecular effects, and many other factors.

Does the body respond differently when blood oxygen saturation is enhanced, or is increased saturation just an indication or response to other actions going on in the body? As mentioned in chapter six, a change was found in 18 proteins resulting from the effects of Tai Chi practice. What other molecular effects are going on in the body during and following Metarobic exercises, and how do the effects of these exercises differ from conventional exercise? The many benefits of Tai Chi have been well documented to various degrees. Aside from more stringent studies more carefully describing and evaluating style, pace, and practice, it is time to begin looking more thoroughly at the underlying causes of these benefits – the physiological changes that occur from Metarobic practice, and how these effects might differ from other forms of exercise.

In time, a growing body of research will determine guidelines for optimal lengths of practice, and which kinds of Metarobic movements are best for various conditions and concerns, as well as for overall health. The mix of Tai Chi with Qi Gong in many scientific studies have made the water muddy as to what exactly is providing the benefits. Most studies mention auxiliary exercises in addition to Tai Chi, which is usually some form of Qi Gong. The question then needs to be asked – are benefits primarily from Tai Chi, the Qi Gong, or both? Since most Tai Chi classes and practice include some form of Qi Gong as well, it may not be a concern. Since both are practiced, a student would get the benefits of both.

In my own practice, I generally begin with four repetitions of the Eight Treasures exercise, followed by 30 minutes or so of Tai Chi. Those people who just do the eight treasures tend to advocate eight to twelve repetitions. When my Tai Chi teacher was asked which exercise would be the most important to practice for health, if a person were to just pick one, he stated the Eight Treasures. Independent study of Tai Chi and forms of Qi Gong may yield some interesting results. As the field grows, adaptations and related forms of movement may come to expand the variety of exercises which fall under the category of Metarobic exercises. Forms of exercises which may come to include forms of walking, Yoga and other exercises which focus on the breath. In the long run, it may be that different forms of Metarobic exercises may yield slightly different benefits, similar to the varied benefits of low and high intensity aerobics.

Conclusion and Future Directions

Metarobics, Tai Chi Therapy and the Beginnings of a New Field of Exercise

It may seem odd in this day and age to think that the categories of fitness we are so familiar with may not explain the benefits for all forms of exercise. Yet when I looked at exercises such as Tai Chi and Qi Gong, I realized that there *had* to be something different going on in the body. That a new and separate field of exercise had to exist. A category which with time may come to include not just Tai Chi and forms of Qi Gong, but also a variety of exercises that do not fit into the traditional aerobic and anaerobic categories. Exercises such as forms of walking and Yoga, or any practice which emphasizes the breath and relaxation, without accelerating the heart rate to aerobic levels.

Tai Chi Cured A Life Dying From Drugs, Alcohol And Sex

T.T. Liang was a well-known teacher and author of several books on Tai Chi, who began learning Tai Chi later in life. He had been living a hard life involving drugs, alcohol and sexual activity, as a government official in Shanghai in the 1940's. Eventually his excessive lifestyle caught up with him, and Liang fell seriously ill and was hospitalized for almost two months. He had developed pneumonia, liver infection and severe gonorrhea. At age 45, his doctors has little hope for his recovery, and gave him about two months to live. Not wanting to die, Liang immediately began learning Tai Chi. Within six months he had recovered most of his health. Reforming his ways, T.T. Liang went on to live to the age of 102 years old, which he attributed to his Tai Chi practice.

From *Victoria Taiji Academy. Grandmaster T.T. Liang.*

Others have observed that walking, if it incorporates a rhythmic stride of the legs and deeper breathing, may have similarities to Qi Gong exercise. Danny and Katherine Dreyer wrote a book about this called *Qi Walking: Fitness Walking for Lifelong Health and Energy.*[1] The way one breaths may be a key element in maximizing the health benefits of walking. The study conducted by Dr. Chetta and colleagues, presented in chapter one, showed that normal walking had little effect on blood oxygen saturation.[2] But when using a pulse oximeter during my own walks, I have found that when I focus on slower diaphragmatic breathing while relaxing any tension in my body, my blood oxygen saturation will usually increase by a percentage point or more.

Walking is considered good for your health, and is classified as a low key and low impact aerobic exercise. But does walking really accelerate the heart rate to levels that will have a large effect on the cardiovascular system, enough to be considered a truly aerobic exercise? In a two year study of 3,208 men and women over the age of 65, researchers found that those in the lower third of walking speed (1.5 miles per hour for men, and 1.35 miles per hour for women) had three times the increased risk of death from cardiovascular disease than did those in the upper third of walking speed (1.85 miles per hour or more for men, and 1.5 miles or more per hour for women).[3] Keep in mind however, that although slower walkers had a higher incidence of death due to cardiovascular disease than faster walkers, the study did not examine any other benefits participants might have received, nor a comparison to those who did not walk at all.

In a study which compared the benefits of Tai Chi, walking, and no exercise (discussed in Chapter Five), benefits where found in the Tai Chi group for COPD, but no change in condition was found in the walking group. The no exercise group experienced a decline in health.[4] So walking did have some benefit, but not to the same degree as did Tai Chi. Which may bring everything back to the breath. Does how one breaths while walking make a difference? And then there is Yoga. How would Yoga fit into the Metarobic perspective?

In my own measurements, the Qi Gong exercise Pa Duan Jin (The Eight Pieces of Silk Brocade, or Eight Treasures) resulted in the largest increase of blood oxygen saturation (two to three percentage points, with highest levels during the standing poses versus the crouching poses). It may be a matter of shades, with forms of Qi Gong one step above Tai Chi, and Tai Chi one step above walking, in relation to Metarobic benefits.

But even here the nature of the movements and breathing seem to be a major factor, at least in relation to blood oxygen saturation. One movement during my Tai Chi practice ("Grasp the Birds' Tail," a series of stationary movements) consistently results in the greatest increase in blood oxygen saturation during the Tai Chi form. Just as there are high and low impact aerobics, there may also be variations in Metarobic exercises.

Ultimately, for total health, it may be important to develop a well-rounded exercise routine, one including aerobic, strength training, stretching, *and* Metarobic exercise. But if health conditions preclude more vigorous forms of exercise at the outset, Metarobic exercises may help enhance health until one is able to engage in a larger variety of exercises. Metarobic exercise provides one more choice, opening up avenues of exercise which can alleviate boredom, match the interests of a diverse population, and provide an additional opportunity relative to current fitness level and ability.

Tai Chi – A "Prescription for Pain, High Blood Pressure, and Diabetes."

"In addition to a number of physical problems (diabetes and high blood pressure), in February 2003, I had a back operation. It was only partially successful. For almost a year I tried physical therapy and medications. Even with ever-increasing dosages of pain medicine, I got little relief. I decided to try Tai Chi. By the third session, I could stand for more than an hour without pain. I didn't need pain medication any longer. When my doctor saw my improvement, he stopped my physical therapy. The doctor asked me what had changed. I told him I was doing T'ai Chi, he said, "If I had known you had access to Tai Chi, I would have told you to start the exercise immediately." He warned me, though, that if I ever stopped, I might regress. In the course of time, my other medical problems went away. I eventually stopped taking medication for my diabetes and high blood pressure. I have also learned to relax and have found some stress relief and a sense of peace – but these are issues that I'm still working on."

- T.S (From *Everyday Tai Chi. Testimonials*).

If deeper abdominal breathing and relaxation are the key factors for Metarobic benefits, then the term may come to encompass many other exercises as well. Over time, the venues which constitute Metarobic exercise may include a surprising number of activities, just as aerobics has expanded to include everything from running to aerobic routines to cardio kickboxing and Zumba.

But as they say, variety is the spice of life, and the new and infant science of Metarobics should be no different. What may attract one person may be unpleasant to another. Tai Chi and related exercises add one more option for health. An option which may become a necessity, if faced with certain health conditions. As my theories and ideas are tested, some may be discarded as outright wrong, others confirmed as on the dot, and new understandings may arise beyond enhanced blood oxygen saturation, diffusion, and metabolic effects. Benefits which can include the psychological, as described below.

Psychological Benefits of Tai Chi

Tai Chi as a mindfulness based activity carries additional benefits for physical and mental health. Mindfulness based practices have long been used to enhance awareness of destructive actions and habits in various Eastern traditions. Self-destructive actions can include not just addictions to smoking, alcohol or other drugs, but can also include poor eating habits, as well as addiction to TV or video games. Enhanced states of mindfulness can increase awareness of how and when you engage in moments of self-sabotage, in personal relationships, as well as in life in general.

Over the past century, the top ten causes of early death have shifted from infectious diseases such as pneumonia and tuberculosis, to diseases caused primarily by lifestyle – primarily related to diet and activity level. So aside from Metarobic benefits for physical health, Metarobic exercises such as Tai Chi carry an additional benefit in the form of enhanced awareness, mindfulness and self-control over what are often unconscious behaviors, including health behavior.

Deaths due to sedentary living accounts for approximately 33% of early deaths (including death from coronary heart disease, colon cancer and diabetes), while lifestyle choices are the primary factor in 75% of all early deaths. These are diseases for which physical activity is established as a causal factor to one degree or another).[5] Obesity is a major risk factor for the development of chronic diseases. The Center for Disease Control (CDC) notes that from 1960 to 2010, adult obesity increased in adults from 13% to 37.5%, and from 5% to 17% in youths 19 and under.[6]

Mindful awareness of eating habits, and what factors drive when and what and where you eat, can lead over time to a better control of diet and even exercise habits. Much of over eating is driven by a stress reaction.[7] Tai Chi can have a direct effect on the stress response through the relaxation factor, as well as through a better awareness and control over stressful situations and what drives them.

Tai Chi has been called "moving meditation," due to mental effects similar to sitting or walking meditation. Focusing on the leading hand during Tai Chi practice is much like using a focal point in Zen meditation, which uses the breath, a mantra, candle or other focal point. By focusing the mind on one point, the ongoing and constant mental chatter that streams through the mind becomes quieted, resulting in a clear mind. Aside from more efficient mental functioning, the calming effect of Tai Chi also helps to deal with stress. Enhanced insight can also help a person gain control over addictions such as smoking.

Although tobacco also has physiological addictive properties, much of smoking habit is just that – habit. Over the years I have had students in my Tai Chi classes who have come up to me at the end of the semester, and told me that they quit smoking because of Tai Chi. This caught me by surprise, considering I had never talked about smoking in any of my classes. One student even told me that before the Tai Chi class, he had never contemplated giving up cigarettes. There was just something about Tai Chi that led him to stop smoking.

Tai Chi, Awareness And Smoking

"First, I realized that when practicing Tai Chi on a regular basis, my cravings were lessened during the day. I'm not sure if this was a physical effect of the relaxed breathing, or if it was psychological. When I went for longer periods of not doing Tai Chi, my cravings increased. I have been wanting to focus on living a healthy lifestyle and maybe doing Tai Chi made me more aware and put my mind in a "healthy" state, because every time I craved a cigarette, I thought to myself, 'that is not healthy.'"

- Paul (From the study on Tai Chi and Smoking Cessation. [8])

All of these students told me that a growing awareness of their smoking habits played a major role in their quitting. I grew curious about this, so I began researching to see if others had similar experiences. In doing so, I found a Tai Chi program specifically targeted at smoking cessation, at the University of Miami. In that study, 83 percent of participants quit smoking as a result of the program.[8]

The responses of the students in my class, as well as a letter describing a participant's experience in the Miami study, indicated that a growing awareness of smoking habits and triggers were a major factor (possibly in conjunction with physiological responses). Enhanced awareness through meditation has been a valuable tool for behavior change for over 2500 years, first in the East, and later in the West. In the West, meditative practices for behavior change have been popularized by Jon Kabat-Zinn as Mindfulness Meditation,[9] as a behavioral intervention aimed at transforming behavior through enhanced nonjudgmental in-the-moment awareness.

Awareness (*Sati* in Pali, an early Indian language still used in Zen and Buddhist studies, due to the origin of these practices) is a major component in Buddhist philosophy, as a means of eliminating destructive behavior and thoughts. Meditation is used as a tool to develop awareness of destructive habits and reactions, to enhance identification of cues triggering negative behavior. A basic premise is that the awareness and identification of cues instigating negative reactions is sufficient for creating awareness of cause and effect, and more importantly, a separation of self from behavior. Essentially a mental "stepping back," allowing space for purposeful action, as opposed to uncontrolled and unconscious reaction.

Without awareness of what needs changing, and of the destructive influence of unconscious negative behaviors and reactions, change will never happen. Even something as obvious as putting a cigarette in your mouth can become an unconscious habit. Awareness of smoking related cues and triggers can develop a conscious control of smoking behavior. One of the nice things about Tai Chi, is that as a moving form of meditation, Tai Chi can be an effective and attractive tool for creating mindful awareness for breaking unconscious habits, with many ancillary health benefits.

To use Tai Chi as a moving form of meditation, it becomes more necessary to be able to practice the form on your own, as opposed to following along using cues provided by a teacher or video. The primary reason for this relates to the focus of the mind during Tai Chi. In sitting meditation, the meditator focuses the mind on the breath, often counting each breath to 10 and then starting over again. Other focal points are also used, but this is one of the most common, particularly for beginners.

When counting the breath, it is common in the beginning stages to lose count of the breath, either continuing past 10, or losing count entirely as other thoughts intrude (such as "I wonder what I will have for lunch today"). Over time, by continually bringing the focus of the mind back to the breath and the 10 count, distracting and rambling thoughts disappear, leaving a calm and tranquil mind. From this calm tranquil mind comes a new level of awareness, an enhanced ability to perceive negative actions and their sources, in yourself and those around you. With enhance awareness comes better communication, as well as self-awareness of destructive behaviors.

    Tai Chi acts in a similar way, but rather than counting the breath, the Tai Chi practitioner places the focus of the mind on the leading hand. As the hand drifts before your face, the mind follows. As the passive hand rises to take the leading hands place, the mind continues to follow, focused on whichever hand takes the lead. Such focus develops over time into a calm tranquility, so much so that even the sensation of time ceases to exist. Thirty minutes of practice will seem to pass in an instant.

    In an older adult Tai Chi class, I have participants focus on developing enhanced awareness of body movements, posture, balance and relaxation, using just one Tai Chi movement (Grasp the Bird's Tail). Class members were amazed the first few times they performed the one movement over and over again, with focus, for over 30 minutes, stating that they had no sensation of the passage of time. It felt like at most only a few minutes had passed.

    Just as incessant thoughts and mental ramblings quiet under the focus of the ten count in sitting meditation, so does the mind by focusing on the movements of Tai Chi. And with this growing mental calm, comes greater self-understanding, insights and awareness. And additional benefit is alleviation from boredom. Some people look at Tai Chi, and feel that moving slowly though the form would be boring. Much of boredom comes from thinking and focusing on time. Being mindful and focused on the movements results in a suspended state beyond time.

Since the focus of Metarobics is on the physiological reactions of the body during Tai Chi and similar exercises, I will go into greater detail regarding the many psychological benefits of Tai Chi in a later book, *Tai Chi – Mind, Body and Spirit*. In that book I will also touch on the more metaphysical aspects of meditative practice, as well as forms of energy work which are popular in some schools of Tai Chi and Qi Gong. As my Tai Chi teacher stated, 90 percent of the time, Qi just means air. But the other 10 percent holds some fascinating implications. Implications already familiar to those who have experienced the runners high, or the spiritual awareness that comes from the many forms of contemplative practice (including forms of Christianity and Zen Buddhism).

Final Thoughts

Long term longitudinal studies of Tai Chi practitioners has been difficult to accomplish, due to the relative limited number of people who engage in these forms of exercise (compared to running and walking). But as these arts become more popular, it will be easier to follow the lives of larger populations, in order to better understand the long term health benefits of Tai Chi and forms of Qi Gong.

As the growing number of Tai Chi practitioners age, more support for the life giving benefits for these exercises will arise, just as the growing number of runners give testimonial to the benefits of that exercise. Tai Chi masters are renowned for their longevity, as well as their health and vitality. Even many of the early masters, who often drank and smoked heavily as part of the culture of the time, still lived well into their 70's and 80's, active and mobile even into old age. Some lived to be over 90 or 100 years of age, including TT Liang who lived to 102, whose story is presented in this chapter. Run Run Shaw, the pioneering Hong Kong movie producer of Kung Fu movies, lived to be 107 years old, which he attributed to a variety of factors, including the practice of Qi Gong.[10]

Tai Chi Therapy – The Science of Metarobics, helps lay a theoretical groundwork for a group of exercises which have already demonstrated so much for so many. This book highlighted research on the effects of hypoxia and Tai Chi for a wide range of chronic conditions. Ultimately the number of conditions Metarobic exercises may benefit may be limitless, since efficient oxygen use is critical for every function in the body, from thinking to healing. Parkinson's and Alzheimer's are but two more areas which were not covered in the preceding chapters, but for which there is evidence that Tai Chi may benefit.[11]

Risk factors that may increase risk of Alzheimer includes lack of exercise, smoking, high blood pressure, high cholesterol, and poorly controlled diabetes.[12] Since Tai Chi is a form of exercise that has been demonstrated to reduce high blood pressure, cholesterol, help control diabetes, and can impact smoking habits, it offers promise as an exercise that may hold off or diminish the effects of Alzheimer's. The action of increased blood diffusion may also offer benefits, since brain cells depend on efficient microcirculation to carry nutrients and other essential materials (including oxygen) throughout the brain. Vascular dementia, another type of cognitive decline which may be linked with Alzheimer's, is caused by damaged blood vessels in the brain, again stressing the importance of good blood circulation in all areas of the body, including the brain.

Factors which may reduce your risk have been identified as participating in mentally challenging leisure activities (such as learning more advanced forms of Tai Chi), and social interactions.[12] Tai Chi is often performed in social groups. One recent study sought to determine potential effects of Tai Chi on brain size and cognition, with possible effects on Alzheimer's disease.[13] Participants in the Tai Chi group were compared to a literature discussion group. Both groups demonstrated a significant increase in brain volume, comparable to previous studies documenting the benefit of aerobic exercise on brain volume. A control group experienced brain shrinkage over the same period typical for the 60 to 70 year age group.

The authors note that gradual cognitive deterioration which precedes dementia is associated with increased shrinkage of the brain, as nerve cells and connections are gradually lost. It is unknown at this point if such activities could help prevent Alzheimer's disease, but the authors state that epidemiological studies have shown that those who engage in regular physical exercise, or are more socially active, have a lower risk of Alzheimer disease. People with Alzheimer's also become more susceptible to falls. As mentioned earlier, the development of enhanced balance is one of the primary hallmarks and benefits of Tai Chi.

Parkinson's disease is also a progressive disorder of the nervous system, that primarily affects movement.[11,14] Beginning stages can include a mild tremor of the hand, slowed motion (including short shuffling steps), rigid muscles, impaired posture and balance, speech changes, and in later stages signs of dementia, similar to Alzheimer's. The causes are unknown, but genetics and environmental factors (i.e. exposure to toxins or certain viruses) are thought to play a role.

If so, then aside from controlling for toxins and viruses, Tai Chi practice may help the body to better deal with viruses (as discussed above in chapter six, in the section on immunity), and may also help through elimination of toxins through enhanced metabolism and removal of wastes. According to the Mayo clinic,[14] maintaining muscle strength and movement can help with some of the progressive tendencies of Parkinson's. Tai Chi, as a mild form of exercise which focuses on stability, balance and movement, may be a particularly suitable form of exercise, and is recommended by the Mayo Clinic.

By scientifically evaluating the actions of the body during Metarobic based exercises, more beneficial and accurate prescription and practice of these exercises will be possible, to the point where Tai Chi and related exercises can be prescribed as effective forms of therapy for many conditions.

Tai Chi Made Me Walk Again

My mom was diagnosed with Parkinson's disease. Her movements were stiff and awkward, and she dragged her feet when trying to walk. Finally she needed a walker, just to shuffle along. Then she started Tai Chi. A year later, my mom's movements improved so much, that not only did she not need the walker, but she could walk completely unaided. Tai Chi made a major difference in her symptoms and quality of life.

Personal account related at a conference.

As with any new theory, use these exercises in a way that makes sense to you, and to your doctor. It is my hope and wish that this book will make understanding and practice a little more clear. Metarobic exercises such as Tai Chi have been used by a large number of people with severe health conditions, with almost miraculous effects.

Having a better understanding of the reasons for these benefits will do nothing to harm the mystique of Tai Chi. But over time, a greater understanding will do much for coming to know how to best maximize the desired benefits. As a new science with an old tradition, Metarobics is just the beginning.

REFERENCES

Preface:

1. Lee MS, Lee E, Ernst E. Is tai chi beneficial for improving aerobic capacity? A systematic review. British Journal of Sports Medicine. 2009 43; 569-573.

2. Cooper K. Aerobics. M Evans distributor, Lippincott, Philadelphia. 1968.

Chapter 1:

1. Cooper K. Aerobics. M Evans distributor, Lippincott, Philadelphia. 1968.

2. Larkey L, Jahnke R, Etnier J, Gonzalez J. Meditative Movement as a Category of Exercise: Implications for Research. Journal of Physical Activity and Health, 2009, 6, 230-238

3. Stock N, Chibon F, Binh MBN, et al. Adult-type rhabdomyosarcoma: analysis of 57 cases with clinicopathologic description, identification of 3 morphologic patterns and prognosis. Am Journal of Surgical Pathology. 2009; 33(12):1850-1859.

4. Yang KD, Chang WC, Chuang H, et al. Increased complement factor H with decreased factor B determined by proteomic differential displays as a biomarker of tai chi chuan exercise. Clinical Chemistry 56:1 (2010) 127-131

5. Gryffin PA. Qi: Implications for a new paradigm of exercise. Integrative Medicine. 2013;12(1):36-40.

6. Mayo Clinic. Hypoxemia. http://www.mayoclinic.org/symptoms/hypoxemia/basics/definition/sym-20050930

7. Wang C, Schwaitzberg S, Berliner E, Zarin DA, Lau J. Hyperbaric oxygen for treating wounds: a systematic review of the literature. Arch Surg. 2003 Mar; 138(3):272-9

8. Oxford Chinese Dictionary. Cambridge: Oxford University Press. 2010

9. Chetta A, Zaninib A, Pisic G, Aielloa M, Tzania P, Nerib M, Olivieria D. Reference values for the 6 minute walk test in healthy subjects 20-50 years old. Respiratory Medicine 2006; 100:1573-1578.

10. Galy O, Hue O, Chamari K, Boussana A, Chaouachi A, Prefaut C (2008). Influence of performance level on exercise-induced arterial hypoxemia during prolonged and successive exercise in triathletes. International Journal of Sports Physiology and Performance; 3: 482-500.

11. Dreyer D, Dreyer K. Qi Walking: Fitness Walking for Lifelong Health and Energy. Touchstone; 2006.

12. Center for Disease Control (CDC). Health, United States, 2010.

www.cdc.gov/nchs/data/hus/hus10.pdf. Updated 2010.

13. Wang C, Schmid C, Kalish R, Yinh J, Rones R, Goldenberg D, McAlindon T. Tai Chi is Effective in Treating Fibromyalgia: A Randomized Controlled Trial. The New England Journal of Medicine. 2010; 363: 743-54.

14. Abbot RB, Hui K, Hays RD, Li M, Pan T. A randomized controlled trial of tai chi for tension headaches. Evidence Based Complement and Alternative Medicine. 2007;12 4(1):107-113.

15. Song R, Lee EO, Lam P, Bae SC. Effects of tai chi exercise on pain, balance, muscle strength, and perceived difficulties in physical functioning in older women with osteoarthritis: a randomized clinical trial. Journal of Rheumatology. 2003;30(9):2039-44.

16. Uhlig T, Fongen C, Steen E, Christie A, Ødegård S. Exploring Tai Chi in rheumatoid arthritis: a quantitative and qualitative study. BMC Musculoskeletal Disorders 2010, 11:43

Testimonials

Elisa "A miracle? No, we say, 'It's the tai chi practice.'" by John Morella www.taichiforhealthinstitute.org/newsletter/individual_newsletter.php?id=180#1

Saundra. Tai Chi for Everyone. Testimonials.
www.taichiforeveryone.net/main/testimonials.htm

Margaret (From Bikram Yoga St. Louis). Testimonials.
http://yogastlouis.com/testimonial/health-benefits-i-never-expected/

Carol. Tai Chi for Health Institute. Newsletters.
www.taichiforhealthinstitute.org/

Solange. Sing Ong Tai Chi. Testimonials.
http://taichi-chuan.org/testimonials/

Chapter 2:

1. Oxford Chinese Dictionary. Cambridge: Oxford University Press, 2010.

2. International Standard Chinese – English Basic Nomenclature of Chinese Medicine. Beijing: People's Medical Publishing House; 2008.

3. Chinese-English Chinese Traditional Medical Word-Ocean Dictionary. Taiyuan: Shanxi Ren Min Chu Ban She; 1995.

4. Gryffin P. Qi: Implications for a new paradigm of exercise. Integr Med. 2013;12(1):36-40.

5. Kbarends. Ki-hanja. Wikipedia.
    http://en.wikipedia.org/wiki/File:Ki-hanja.png.

Released into the public domain by the author, without any conditions. 2006

6. Zhang YH, Rose K. A brief history of qi. Paradigm Publications, MA, 2001.

7. Jahnke R. The Healing Promise of Qi. McGraw Hill Books, NY. 2002

8. Lowenthal W. There are No Secretes: Professor Cheng Man Ch'ing and His T'ai Chi Chuan. Blue Snake Books. 1993

9. Medline Plus U.S. National Library of Medicine. Aging Changes in Organs. www.nlm.nih.gov/medlineplus/ency/article/004012.htm

10. Elliot WJ, Izzo JL. Device-Guided Breathing to Lower Blood Pressure: Case Report and Clinical Overview. MedGenMed. 2006; 8(3): 23.

11. Bernardi L1, Spadacini G, Bellwon J, Hajric R, Roskamm H, Frey AW. Effect of breathing rate on oxygen saturation and exercise performance in chronic heart failure. Lancet. 1998. 351(9112):1308-11.

Testimonials

Ramel Rones. Tai Chi and Qi Gong for Health and Wellness. http://ramelrones.com/blog/2013/4/3/rick-abrams-10-year-thyroid-cancer-journey-and-tai-chi

Finding My Way Back from a Near Death by Ted Saji. www.taichiforhealthinstitute.org/newsletter/individual_newsletter.php?id=205#ted

Chapter 3:

1. Pederson PL. Warburg, me and hexokinase 2: multiple discoveries of key molecular events underlying one of cancers' most common phenotypes, the "Warburg effect". i.e. Elevated glycolysis in the presence of oxygen. Journal of Bioenergetics and Biomembranes 2007;39:211-222.

2. Maleki T, Cao N, Song S, Kao C, Ko SC, Ziaie B. An ultrasonically-powered implantable micro oxygen generator (IMOG). IEEE Transactions Biomedical Engineering Journal; 2011; 58(11): 3104-3111.

3. Benito J, Shi Y, Szymanska B, Carol H, Boehm I, et al. (2011) Pronounced Hypoxia in Models of Murine and Human Leukemia: High Efficacy of Hypoxia-Activated Prodrug PR-104. PLoS ONE 6(8): e23108. doi: 10.1371/journal.pone.0023108

4. Wilson WR1, Hay MP. Targeting hypoxia in cancer therapy. Nat Rev Cancer. 2011 Jun;11(6):393-410. doi: 10.1038/nrc3064

5. Brahimi-Horn MC, Chiche J, Pouyssegur J. Hypoxia and cancer. Journal of Molecular Medicine; 2007; 85:1301-1307

6. Xue M, Kong, FM, Yu, J. Implementation of hypoxia measurement into lung cancer therapy. Lung Cancer;2012; 75: 146-150.

7. Zitta K, Meybohm P, Albrecht M, et al. Salicylic acid induces apoptosis in colon carcinoma cells grown in-vitro: Influence of oxygen and salicylic acid concentration. Experimental Cell Research. 2012; 318(7):828-834.

8. Tavers J, Dudgeon DJ, Amjadi K, et al. Mechanisms of exertional dyspnea in patients with cancer. Journal of Applied Physiology. 2007;104:57-66.

9. Nieto FJ, Peppard PE, Young T, et al. Sleep-disordered breathing and cancer mortality: results from the Wisconsin Sleep Cohort Study. American Journal of Respiratory and Critical Care Medicine. 2012; 186(2) 190-194.

10. Stock N, Chibon F, Binh MBN, et al. Adult-type rhabdomyosarcoma: analysis of 57 cases with clinicopathologic description, identification of 3 morphologic patterns and prognosis. Am Journal of Surgical Pathology. 2009; 33(12):1850-1859.

11. Zeng Y, Luo T, Xie H, Huang M, Cheng A. Health benefits of qigong or tai chi for cancer patients: a systematic review and meta-analyses. Complement Ther Med. 2014 Feb;22(1):173-86.

12. Sprod LK1, Janelsins MC, Palesh OG, et al. Health-related quality of life and biomarkers in

breast cancer survivors participating in tai chi chuan. Journal Cancer Surviv. 2012 Jun;6(2):146-54.

13. Roxburgh CS, McMillan DC. Cancer and systemic inflammation: treat the tumour and treat the host. British Journal of Cancer (2014) 110, 1409–1412.

14. Palasuwan A, Suksom D, Margaritis I, Soogarun S, Rousseau A. Effects of Tai Chi Training on Antioxidant Capacity in Pre- and Postmenopausal Women. Journal of Aging Research. 2011

15. Kuender D. Yang, Wan-Ching Chang, Hau Chuang, Pei-Wen Wang, Rue-Tsuan Liu, Shu-Hui Yeh. Increased complement factor H with decreased factor B determined by proteomic differential displays as a biomarker of tai chi chuan exercise. Clinical Chemistry 56:1 (2010) 127-131

16. Smith D, Russell F. The Healing Journey: The Odyssey of an Uncommon Athlete. Random House, 1984.

Testimonials

Burr M. Opening And Closing The Gates Of Heaven: Helen Liang's Triumph Over Tragedy, Battling Lymphoma With Qigong, Tai Chi And Chinese Medicine. Kung Fu Tai Chi Magazine. 2003 July/August.

http://www.kungfumagazine.com/magazine/article.php?article=353

David. Cancer Active. Tai Chi the Energy Within. www.canceractive.com/cancer-active-page-link.aspx?n=472

Pike G. The Power of Qi. Bell Publishing Company. 1981

Cristela Gutierrez. The Seventh Happiness School of Chi Gong. www.masterteresa.com/testimonials.html#cancer

Unknown. Faulk Tai Chi. Testimonials. www.faulktaichi.com/testimonials/

Bhavna. The Health Site. http://www.thehealthsite.com/news/yoga-therapy-can-cure-every-disease-even-cancer/

Huixian. The Experience Project. http://www.experienceproject.com/stories/Practice-Qi-Gong/500558

Karyn. Spring Forest Qi Gong Testimonials. http://www.springforestqigong.com/index.php/testimonials

Chapter 4:

1. American Hospital Association. Are Medicare Patients Getting Sicker?

www.aha.org/research/reports/tw-ptacuity.pdf

2. CDC. Heart disease facts. http://www.cdc.gov/heartdisease/facts.htm

3. Li J, Thorne LN, Pnjabi NM, et al. Intermittent hypoxia induces hyperlipidemia in lean mice. Circulation Research. 2005 97(7): 698-706.

4. Yamamoto K, Kawano H, Gando Y, et al. Poor trunk flexibility is associated with arterial stiffening. American Journal of Physiology - Heart and Circulatory Physiology. 2009 (297): H1314-H1318

5. American Heart Association. Stress and Blood Pressure. http://www.heart.org/HEARTORG/Conditions/HighBloodPressure/PreventionTreatmentofHighBloodPressure/Stress-and-Blood-Pressure_UCM_301883_Article.jsp

6. Michels KB, Rosner BA, Manson JE, et al. Prospective Study of Calcium Channel Blocker Use, Cardiovascular Disease, and Total Mortality Among Hypertensive Women Circulation. 1998; 97: 1540-1548

7. National Stroke Association. Stroke Prevention. http://www.stroke.org/site/PageServer?pagename=prevent

8. Sung BH, Joseph L. Izzo JL, Wilson MF. Effects of Cholesterol Reduction on BP Response to Mental Stress in Patients with High

Cholesterol. American Journal of Hypertension. 1997; 10(6): 592-599

9. American Heart Association. Ischemic Strokes (Clots). http://www.strokeassociation.org/STROKEORG/AboutStroke/TypesofStroke/IschemicClots/Ischemic-Strokes-Clots_UCM_310939_Article.jsp

10. American Heart Association. Hemorrhagic Strokes: Bleeds. http://www.strokeassociation.org/STROKEORG/AboutStroke/TypesofStroke/HemorrhagicBleeds/Hemorrhagic-Strokes-Bleeds_UCM_310940_Article.jsp

11. American Heart Association. Kidney Damage and High Blood Pressure. http://www.heart.org/HEARTORG/Conditions/HighBloodPressure/WhyBloodPressureMatters/Kidney-Damage-and-High-Blood-Pressure_UCM_301825_Article.jsp

12. Nangaku M. Chronic Hypoxia and Tubulointerstitial Injury: A Final Common Pathway to End-Stage Renal Failure. Journal of the American Society of Nephrology. 2006; 17(1): 17-25

13. Haase VH. Hypoxia-inducible factor signaling in the development of kidney fibrosis. Fibrogenesis Tissue Repair. 2012; 6;5 Suppl 1:S16

14. Nangaku M, Rosenberger C, Heyman SN, Eckardt K. Regulation of hypoxia-inducible

factor in kidney disease. Clinical and Experimental Pharmacology and Physiology. 2013; 40 (2): 148–157

15. Palm F, Nordquist L. Renal Tubulointerstitial Hypoxia: Cause and Consequence of Kidney Dysfuction. Clinical and Experimental Pharmacology and Physiology. 2011; 38(7): 424–430.

16. Legrand M, Mik EG, Johannes T, Payen D, Ince C. Renal Hypoxia and Dysoxia After Reperfusion of the Ischemic Kidney. Molecular Medicine. 2008; 14(7-8): 502–516.

17. Yeh GY, Wang C, Wayne PM, Phillips R. Tai chi exercise for patients with cardiovascular conditions and risk factors: A systematic review. Journal of Cardiopulmonary Rehabilitation and Prevention. 2009;29(3):152-160.

18. Yeh G, Wang C, Wayne P, Philips R. The effect of tai chi exercise on blood pressure: A systematic review. Preventive Cardiology. 2008;11(2):82-89.

19. Sato S, Makita S, Uchida R, Ishihara S, Masuda M. Effect of Tai Chi training on baroreflex sensitivity and heart rate variability in patients with coronary heart disease. International Heart Journal. 2010; 51(4):238-41.

20. Ng SM, Wang CW, Ho RT, Ziea TC, He J, Wong VC, Chan CL. Tai chi exercise for patients with

heart disease: a systematic review of controlled clinical trials. Alternative Therapies in Health and Medicine. 2012; 18(3):16-22.

21. Thornton EW, Sykes KS, Tang WK. Health benefits of Tai Chi exercise: improved balance and blood pressure in middle-aged women. Health Promotion International. 2004; 19(1):33-8.

22. Ding M. Tai Chi for stroke rehabilitation: a focused review. American Journal of Physical Medicine and Rehabilitation. 2012; 91(12):1091-1096.

Testimonials

Natalie. Tai Chi for Life Online Magazine. Testimonials Tai Chi form, page 1. www.taichiacademy.com.au/magazine/testimonial1

Marilyn. Heart Healthy Living. Reduce Blood Pressure with Tai Chi by Suzanne Wellman. http://www.hearthealthyonline.com/blood-pressure/lower-blood-pressure/tai-chi-reduces-blood-pressure_1.html

James. Tai Chi Fitness for Health. www.tai-chi-fitness-for-health.com/tai-chi-health-healing-evidence.html

Luo Ji-Hong. A Life Through Tai Chi. www.taichi.ca/publications/LuoJiHong.htm

Bob. Tai Chi Chih. What Others Are Saying. https://commonground.episcopalatlanta.org/Content/What_Others_Are_Saying.asp

Mrs. B. Kungfumagazine.com. Tai Chi as Medicine. www.ezine.kungfumagazine.com/forum/showthread.php?t=50553&page=2

Chapter 5:

1. American Lung Association. Chronic Obstructive Pulmonary Disease (COPD) Fact Sheet. www.lung.org/lung-disease/copd/resources/facts-figures/COPD-Fact-Sheet.html

2. CDC. Asthma in the US. www.cdc.gov/vitalsigns/asthma/

3. Gryffin PA, Chen WC. Implications of T'ai chi for smoking cessation. Journal of Alternative and Complementary Medicine. 2013;19(2):141-145.

4. Wang C, Collet JP, Lau J. The effect of Tai Chi on health outcomes in patients with chronic conditions: a systematic review. Arch Intern Med. 2004 Mar 8; 164(5):493-501.

5. Chan AW; Lee A; Suen LK; Tam WW. Tai chi Qigong improves lung functions and activity tolerance in COPD clients: A single blind, randomized controlled trial. Complementary Therapies in Medicine. 2011; 19 (1): 3-11

6. Chang YF, Yang YH, Chen CC, Chiang BL. Tai Chi Chuan training improves the pulmonary function of asthmatic children. Journal of Microbiology, Immunology and Infection. 2008;41(1):88-95.

7. Kiatboonsri S, Vickers E. Effects of Tai Chi Qigong training on exercise performance and airway inflammation in moderate to severe persistent asthma. CHEST Journal Meeting Abstracts 2007; 134(4).

8. Waddell, JA, Emerson PA, Gunstone RF. Hypoxia in bronchial asthma. American Journal of Physiology - Lung Cellular and Molecular Physiology. 2012; 302(5): L455–L462.

9. Kent BD, Mitchell PD, McNicholas WT. Hypoxemia in patients with COPD: cause, effects, and disease progression. International Journal of Chronic Obstructive Pulmonary Disorders. 2011; 6: 199–208.

10. Reuther I, Aldridge D. Qigong Yangsheng as a complementary therapy in the management of asthma: a single-case appraisal. J Altern Complement Med. 1998;4(2):173-83.

Testimonials

Kenneth G. ChiArts.com. Asthma Treated with Qi Gong and Posture Training. www.chi-arts.com/home/74.html?task=view

Walter. Energy Arts. Taoist Breathing for Tai Chi and Meditation

www.energyarts.com/store/products/breathing/t
aoist-breathing-qigong-meditation-cd

Karl. Mindful Tai Chi. Testimonials. www.mindful-taichi.co.uk/testimonials.html

Chris. Tai Chi for Health Institute. Tai Ci for Health Forums. www.taichiforhealthinstitute.org/forums/archive/index.php?t-1767.html

Chapter 6:

1. CDC. Influenza Update for Geriatricians and Other Clinicians Caring for People 65 and Older. http://www.cdc.gov/flu/professionals/2012-2013-guidance-geriatricians.htm

2. Lee AK, Hester RB, Coggin JH, Gottlieb SF. Increased Oxygen Tensions Influence Subset Composition of the Cellular Immune System in Aged Mice. Cancer Biotherapy. 1994; 9(1): 39-54.

3. Yang Y, Verkuilen J, Rosengren KS, Mariani RA, Reed M, Grubisich SA, Woods JA. Effects of a Taiji and Qigong intervention on the antibody response to influenza vaccine in older adults. American Journal of Chinese Medicine. 2007; 35(4):597-607.

4. Robbins JR, Lee SM, Filipovich AH, Szigligeti P, et al. Hypoxia modulates early events in T cell receptor-mediated activation in human T

lymphocytes via Kv1.3 channels. The Journal of Physiology. 2005; 564(Pt 1): 131–143.

5. Yeh, S., Chuang, H., Lin, L., Hsiao, C. & Eng, H. (2006). Regular tai chi exercise enhances functional mobility and CD4CD25 regulatory T cells. British Journal of Sports Medicine, 40, 239-243.

6. Irwin MR, Pike JL, Cole JC, et al. Effects of a Behavioral Intervention, Tai Chi Chih, on Varicella-Zoster Virus Specific Immunity and Health Functioning in Older Adults. Psychosomatic Medicine, 2003; 65(5): 824-830

7. Tamai K, Yamazaki T, Chino T, et al. PDGFRa-positive cells in bone marrow are mobilized by high mobility group box 1 (HMGB1) to regenerate injured epithelia. Proceedings of the National Academy of Science USA 2011; 108: 6609-6614.

8. National Diabetes Information Clearinghouse (NDIC). Causes of Diabetes. http://diabetes.niddk.nih.gov/dm/pubs/causes/

9. American Diabetes Association. Diabetes Basics http://www.diabetes.org/diabetes-basics/prevention/pre-diabetes/

10. U.S. Department of Health and Human Services. National Diabetes Information Clearinghouse (NDIC) http://diabetes.niddk.nih.gov/dm/pubs/overview/

11. Nyengaard JR, Ido Y, Kilo C, Williamson JR. Interactions Between Hyperglycemia and Hypoxia: Implications for Diabetic Retinopathy Diabetes. 2004; 53(11): 2931-2938

12. Heather LC, Clarke K. Metabolism, hypoxia and the diabetic heart. Journal of Molecular and Cellular Cardiology. 2011; 50(4):598-605.

13. Moritz W, Meier F, Stroka DM, Giuliani M, Kugelmeier P, Nett PC, Lehmann R, Candinas D, Gassmann M, Weber M. Apoptosis in hypoxic human pancreatic islets correlates with HIF-1alpha expression. FASEB Journal. 2002;16(7):745-7.

14. Grotenhermen F. Cannabinoids. Current Drug Targets - CNS & Neurological Disorders. 2005 Oct;4(5):507-30.

15. Kuender D. Yang, Wan-Ching Chang, Hau Chuang, Pei-Wen Wang, Rue-Tsuan Liu, Shu-Hui Yeh. Increased complement factor H with decreased factor B determined by proteomic differential displays as a biomarker of tai chi chuan exercise. Clinical Chemistry 56:1 (2010) 127-131

16. Mayo Clinic. Claudication. http://www.mayoclinic.com/health/claudication/DS01052

17. Noël-Jorand MC, Bragard D, Plaghki L. Pain Perception under Chronic High-altitude Hypoxia European Journal of Neuroscience. 1996; 8(10):2075–2079

18. Wang C, Schmid C, Kalish R, Yinh J, Rones R, Goldenberg D, McAlindon T. Tai Chi is Effective in Treating Fibromyalgia: A Randomized Controlled Trial. The New England Journal of Medicine. 2010; 363: 743-54.

19. Abbot RB, Hui K, Hays RD, Li M, Pan T. A randomized controlled trial of tai chi for tension headaches. Evidence Based Complement and Alternative Medicine. 2007;12 4(1):107-113.

20. Song R, Lee EO, Lam P, Bae SC. Effects of tai chi exercise on pain, balance, muscle strength, and perceived difficulties in physical functioning in older women with osteoarthritis: a randomized clinical trial. Journal of Rheumatology. 2003;30(9):2039-44.

21. National Institute of Arthritis and Musculoskeletal and Skin Diseases. Handout on Health: Rheumatoid Arthritis http://www.niams.nih.gov/health_info/Rheumatic_Disease/default.asp

22. Uhlig T, Fongen C, Steen E, Christie A, Ødegård S. Exploring Tai Chi in rheumatoid arthritis: a quantitative and qualitative study. BMC Musculoskeletal Disorders 2010, 11:43

23. PubMed Health. Multiple Sclerosis. http://www.ncbi.nlm.nih.gov/pubmedhealth/PMH0001747/

24. Husted C, Pham L, Hekking A, Niederman R. Improving quality of life for people with chronic conditions: The example of T'ai chi and multiple

sclerosis. Alternative Therapies in Health and Medicine. 1999; 5(5):70-74

25. Mills N, Allen J, Carey Morgan S. Does Tai Chi/Qi Gong help patients with Multiple Sclerosis? Journal of Bodywork and Movement Therapies. 2000: 4(1), 39-48.

Testimonials

Wendy. Wendys Wellness Website. www.wendyswellness.ca/?page_id=54

Bruce. Tai Chi for Health Institute. What Inspired Me to Start Tai Chi. www.taichiforhealthinstitute.org/articles/individual_article.php?id=317

Steve. Orange County Ta Chi Studio. What Our Tai Chi Students Say. www.octaichi.com/tai-chi-testimonials.html

Sharon. Dr Lam's Tai Chi, Health & Lifestyle Newsletter - Issue Number 123, November 2011What Tai Chi Means to Me. www.taichiforhealthinstitute.org/newsletter/individualnewsletter.php?id=519#sharon

Cheryl. Tai Chi for Health Institute. What Inspired Me to Start Tai Chi. http://www.taichiforhealthinstitute.org/articles/individual_article.php?id=317

Heather. Rosewell Tai Chi. Testimonials. www.roswelltaichi.com/Testimonials.html

Neva. Tai Chi for Everyone. Testimonials. www.taichiforeveryone.net/main/testimonials.html

Chapter 7:

1. Wile, D. Taijiquan and Taoism from Religion to Martial Art and Martial Art to Religion. Journal of Asian Martial Arts. 2007;16 (4): 8-45

2. Henning, S. Ignorance, Legend and Taijiquan. Journal of the Chen Style Taijiquan Research Association of Hawaii. 1994; 2 (3): 1-7.

3. Lungs. Innerbody. http://www.innerbody.com/anatomy/respiratory/lungs

4. Wang C, Schmid CH, Hibberd PL, et al. Tai Chi is Effective in Treating Knee Osteoarthritis: A Randomized Controlled Trial. Arthritis and Rheumatology.2009; 61(11): 1545–1553.

5. Hall AM1, Maher CG, Lam P, Ferreira M, Latimer J. Tai chi exercise for treatment of pain and disability in people with persistent low back pain: a randomized controlled trial. Arthritis Care Res (Hoboken). 2011;63(11):1576-83

6. Gryffin, PA Service providers and the KAP Gap: A survey of major tai chi programs in the United States. In Review.

7. Lam P. Teaching tai chi effectively. Tai Chi Productions. 2011

8. Abdullah S, Dar LM, Rashid A, Tewari A. Hirudotherapy /Leech therapy: Applications and Indications in Surgery. Arch Clin Exp Surg. 2012; 1(3): 172-110.

9. Smith D, Russell F. The Healing Journey: The Odyssey of an Uncommon Athlete. Random House, 1984

10. CDC. Falls among older adults: An overview. http://www.cdc.gov/homeandrecreationalsafety/falls/adultfalls.html

11. Frye B, Scheinthal S, Kemarskaya T, Pruchno R. Tai chi and low impact exercise: Effects on the physical functioning and psychological well-being of older people. J Applied Geront. 2007;26(5):433-453.

Testimonials

Dr. Paul Lam. Tai Chi for Health Institute. www.taichiforhealthinstitute.org/print_article.php?id=317

Victoria. Tai Chi Chuan Center. Testimonials. www.taichichuancenter.org/Testimonial.html

Joyce. Tai Chi for Health Institute. www.taichiforhealthinstitute.org/

Lun. Tai Chi Chuan Center. Testimonials Lun Wong. www.taichichuancenter.org/Testimonial.html

Debbie. Tampa Bay Times. www.tampabay.com/news/health/tai-chi-instructor-says-movements-eased-her-pain-asthma/2118619

Jou Tsung Hwa. Taichifarm.org. The Grandmaster. www.taichifarm.org/Grandmaster_Jou_Tsung_hwa.htm

Conclusion and Future Directions

1. Dreyer D, Dreyer K. Qi Walking: Fitness Walking for Lifelong Health and Energy. Touchstone; 2006.

2. Chetta A, Zaninib A, Pisic G, Aielloa M, Tzania P, Nerib M, Olivieria D. Reference values for the 6 minute walk test in healthy subjects 20-50 years old. Respiratory Medicine 2006; 100:1573-1578.

3. Dumurgier J, Elbaz A, Ducimetière P, Tavernier B, Alpérovitch A, Tzourio C. Slow walking speed and cardiovascular death in well-functioning older adults: prospective cohort study. BMJ Open Respiratory Research. 2009; 339

4. Chan AW; Lee A; Suen LK; Tam WW. Tai chi Qigong improves lung functions and activity tolerance in COPD clients: A single blind, randomized controlled trial. Complementary Therapies in Medicine. 2011; 19 (1): 3-11

5. Powell KE, Blair SN. The public health burdens of sedentary living habits: theoretical but realistic estimates. Medicine and Science in Sports and Exercise.1994;26(7):851-6.

6. CDC. Adult Obesity Facts. http://www.cdc.gov/obesity/data/adult.html

7. Harvard Mental Health Letter. Why stress causes people to overeat. http://www.health.harvard.edu/newsletters/Harvard_Mental_Health_Letter/2012/February/why-stress-causes-people-to-overeat

8. Gryffin PA, Chen WC. Implications of T'ai chi for smoking cessation. Journal of Alternative and Complementary Medicine. 2013;19(2):141-145.

9. Kabat-Zinn J. Full catastrophe living: how to cope with stress, pain and illness using mindfulness meditation. Piatkus, 1996

10. Ching, G. Kung Fu Tai Chi Magazine. Obituaries. May June 1994.

11. Klien, PJ. Tai Chi Chuan in the Management of Parkinson's Disease and Alzheimer's Disease. Medicine and Sports Science. 2008; 52:173-81.

12. Mayo Clinic. Alzheimer's Disease. http://www.mayoclinic.com/health/alzheimers-disease/DS00161/DSECTION=causes

13. Mortimer JA, Ding D, Borenstein AR, et al. Changes in brain volume and cognition in a

randomized trial of exercise and social interaction in a community-based sample of non-demented chinese elders. J Alzheimer's Dis. 2012;30(4):757-766.

14. Mayo Clinic. Parkinson's Disease. http://www.mayoclinic.org/diseases-conditions/parkinsons-disease/basics/definition/con-20028488

Testimonials

Grandmaster T.T. Liang. Victoria Taiji Academy. www.chentaichi.org/ttliang.php

T.S. Every day Tai Chi. Testimonials. www.everydaytcc.com/testimonials.htm

Gryffin P. Essential Tai Chi. www.sites.google.com/site/essentialtaichi/

Made in the USA
San Bernardino, CA
18 December 2016